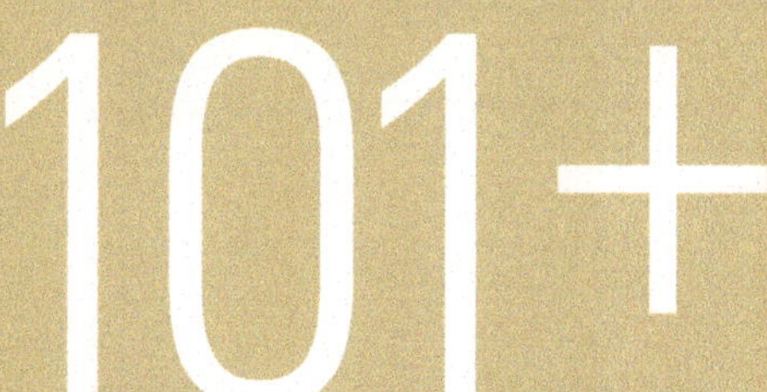

PRIMARY CARE CASE STUDIES

Sampath ("Sam") Wijesinghe, DHSc, MS, MPAS, PA-C, AAHIVS, is an associate professor, director of career development, and associate director of clerkship education at Stanford University School of Medicine's MSPA program. He completed his PA education at Union College, where he received a master's degree in PA studies. He also has a master's degree in management information systems from the University of Nebraska and a doctor of health science degree with an emphasis in global health from A.T. Still University. Dr. Wijesinghe completed an HIV clinical fellowship at University of California San Francisco, Fresno. He has been an HIV specialist since 2014 and has worked in primary care medicine since 2010. He has been involved in medical education since 2013. His clinical interests include primary care medicine, HIV medicine, and global health.

Dr. Wijesinghe practices primary care medicine at Copeland Medical Healthcare Partners, Clovis, California. He practices HIV medicine at Adventist Health Medical Center, Fowler, a small town in California.

Dr. Wijesinghe is committed to educating the next generation of clinicians. With extensive experience in primary care and HIV medicine in underserved areas, he views medical education as an opportunity to improve patient outcomes and advance the field. As a nationally recognized expert, he serves as a CDC clinical ambassador for the Let's Stop HIV Together campaign. In 2023, the Excellence in Partnering award was given to the Together Clinical Ambassador activities, receiving commendable recognition from the CDC Division of HIV Prevention. The Together team extends sincere gratitude to Dr. Wijesinghe for his critical role in training PAs and emerging students, alongside public health clinicians. Additionally, his significant contributions to the medical field through various publications are greatly appreciated. That same year, he was honored as the William H. Marquardt Community Health Access Fellow by the PA Foundation for inspiring both current and aspiring clinicians to engage in underserved areas and address healthcare disparities. A highly sought-after speaker and lecturer, Dr. Wijesinghe has presented at several national conferences and events and educates the next generation of PAs as a clinical preceptor on a regular basis.

Dr. Wijesinghe lives with his wife, Nuwan, and has two children, Rynee and Ryler.

101+

SECOND EDITION

PRIMARY CARE CASE STUDIES

A Workbook for Clinical and Bedside Skills

Sampath Wijesinghe, DHSc, MS, MPAS, PA-C, AAHIVS

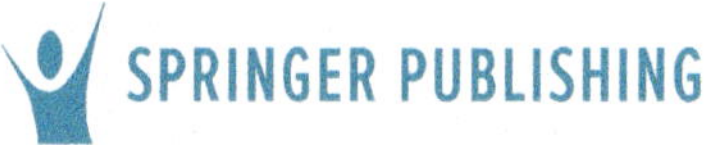

First Springer Publishing edition 978-0-8261-8272-2 (2021)

Springer Publishing Company, LLC
902 Carnegie Center/Suite 140
Princeton, NJ 08540
www.springerpub.com
connect.springerpub.com

Acquisitions Editor: Joseph Morita
Content Development Editor: Julia Curcio
Production Editor: Diana Osborne
Compositor: Amnet

ISBN: 978-0-8261-3967-2
e-book ISBN: 978-0-8261-3968-9
DOI: 10.1891/9780826139689

SUPPLEMENTS:

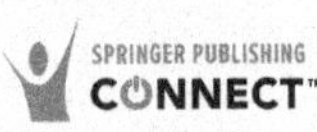

A robust set of instructor resources designed to supplement this text is located at http://connect.springerpub.com/content/book/978-0-8261-3968-9. Qualifying instructors may request access by emailing textbook@springerpub.com.

Instructor Materials:
LMS Common Cartridge–All Instructor Resources ISBN: 978-0-8261-9224-0
Online-Only Cases ISBN: 978-0-8261-3969-6
Instructor Table of Contents ISBN: 978-0-8261-5071-4

25 26 27 / 5 4 3 2

Library of Congress Control Number: 2024042945

Printed in the United States of America.

DEDICATION

To my mentor, Alex Moir (1962–2015), who taught me true compassion and was a mentor and role model beyond compare. It was always my dream that we'd coauthor this book, but that dream could not come true. The world lost a fine man, who could have taught compassion and competent care to generations of future clinicians.

To my parents, David (1944–2015) and Rita Wijesinghe. When I was growing up, our family did not have much, but my parents' unconditional love and fight to provide a better future for me and my loving sister Mangali laid a solid foundation for our journeys. Importantly, my parents always believed in me. I love you more!

To my wife, Nuwan. Meeting you in high school was the best thing that ever happened to me. Marrying you was the best decision I ever made. Everything I do personally or professionally is possible because you are in my life. I love you more than you can imagine.

To my children, Rynee and Ryler. Throughout the preparation of this book, you both selflessly gave me the space and time I needed. I know I have taken too much time away from you because of this publication. Your love and support from the beginning to end has meant the world to me. You two are the reason I want to contribute and make the world a better place!

To medical educators, PAs, NPs, physicians, and future clinicians. For those who practice medicine with the belief that clinical and compassionate skills are equally essential, I extend my heartfelt appreciation. Your enduring commitment to exemplifying these values in your practice, even after many years, inspires me. I dedicate this book to each of you.

CONTENTS

CONTRIBUTORS

Adnaan Edun, MD
Medical Director
Core Faculty
Adventist Health Tulare Rural Health Clinic
Tulare, California

Cherilyn M. Hendrix, DHEd, MSBME, PA-C, DFAAPA
Assistant Dean for Physician Assistant Education
PA Program Director
Associate Professor
University of Maryland Baltimore School of Graduate Studies
Baltimore, Maryland

Amanda J. Ingalls, DMS, PA-C
Director of Didactic Education
Professor of Practice
Keck Graduate Institute
Claremont, California

Shruti Javali, MD
Program Director
Adventist Health Hanford and Sonora Family Medicine Residency Program
Hanford, California

Jason Kessler, MD, FAAP, CMQ
Pediatrician
Primary Health Care, Inc.
Des Moines, Iowa
Medical Director
WPS
Madison, Wisconsin

Emily Lane, MS, APRN, FNP-C
NP Guide, LLC
Anderson, South Carolina

Saul Antonio Diaz Martinez, MD, FAAP
Pediatric Service Line Medical Director
Adventist Health
Fowler, California
Clinical Preceptor
Stanford School of Medicine
Stanford, California
Clinical Assistant Professor Specialty Medicine
California Health Sciences University
Clovis, California

Courtney Reinisch, DNP, RN, FNP-BC, DCC
Professor
School of Nursing
Montclair State University
Montclair, New Jersey

Caroline Rhéaume, MD, MSc, PhD, FCFP, CCFP, DipIBLM, DipABLM
Associate Professor
Family Medicine and Emergency Department
Faculty of Medicine
Université Laval
Quebec City, Québec, Canada

Benjamin Silverberg, MD, MSc, FAAFP, FCUCM
Associate Professor
Division of Ambulatory Operations, Department of Emergency Medicine
Medical Director
Division of Physician Assistant Studies
Department of Human Performance
West Virginia University School of Medicine
Morgantown, West Virginia

Christine Smith, MSN, FNP-C
Family Nurse Practitioner
Peak Medical & Wellness Center
Anthem, Arizona

Linda Takvorian, FNP-C, MSN, RN, CNN
School of Health Professions
National University
Los Angeles, California

Anne Walsh, PA-C, MMSc, DFAAPA
Clinical Professor, PA Studies
Crean College of Health and Behavioral Sciences
Chapman University
Irvine, California

Jennifer Weeks, DNP, FNP-C
Nurse Practitioner
MedNow
Evans, Georgia

Sampath Wijesinghe, DHSc, MS, MPAS, PA-C, AAHIVS
Clinical Associate Professor
Director of Career Development
Associate Director of Clerkship Education
MSPA Studies
Stanford School of Medicine
Primary Care PA-C and HIV Specialist
Copeland Medical Healthcare Partners
Clovis, California

Contributors to the Previous Edition

Valerie Berry, MD

Michael S. Burney, EdD, MS, PA-C

Michael Castillo, MD

Rachel Chappell, MHSc, PA-C

Mark P. Christiansen, PhD, PA-C

Dolores Davis, RN, FNP APRN-C

David Duensing, DO

Christopher P. Forest, DHSc, DFAAPA, PA-C

Tosi Gilford, MD, PA-C

Nancy Hamler, DMSc, MPA, RDN, PA-C

Surani Hayre-Kwan, MBA, DNP, FNP-BC, FACHE, FAANP

Cherilyn M. Hendrix, DHEd, MSBME, PA-C, DFAAPA

Lisa Hood, DNP, MSN, RN, FNP-C

Michael J. Huckabee, PhD, MPAS, PA-C

Amanda J. Ingalls, MS, PA-C

Johnny Jimenez, MSN, APRN, FNP-C

Paramjit Kaur, MSN, FNP-C

Gerald Kayingo, PhD, MMSc, PA-C

Jason R. Kessler, MD, FAAP

Vasco Deon Kidd, DHSc, MPH, MS, PA-C

Timothy Kuntz, MPAS, PA-C

Aimee Larson, MSPA, PA-C

Susan LeLacheur, DrPH, PA-C

Kristy Luciano, MS, PA-C

Erin N. Lunn, PA-C, MHS

Hema Majeno, PA-C

David Malebranche, MD, MPH

April H. Martin, MSPAS, PA-C

Mario Martinez, MD

Lynn H. McComas, DNP, ANP-C, PHN

Kameko Hazley McGuire, DNP, PMHNP-BC, NP-C, RN

Jennifer Momen, MD, MPH, FAAP

Michael N. Moya, MD

Andrew Nevins, MD

Karen Paolinelli, MSN, APRN, FNP-C, PA-C, DFAAPA

Shantha Parameswaran, MD, FAAP

Tushar M. Patel, MD

Jason Radke, MMS, PA-C

Jennifer Ramos, MPAP, PA-C

Karla Reinhart DNP, FNP-C, ARNP

Sara Rygol, MPAS, PA-C

Alfred M. Sadler Jr., MD, FACP, ScD (Hon)

Anabel Segovia, RN, MSN, FNP-C

Tana Summers, MS, PA-C

Laura L. Van Auker, DNP, APRN, FNP-BC, MSN, SN-C

James Van Rhee, MS, PA-C

Veronica Vo, MPAC, PA-C

Anne Walsh, PA-C, MMSc, DFAAPA

Ariel L. Watriss, MSN, NP-C

Jennifer C. Weeks, DNP, FNP-C

REVIEWERS

Camille Bloom, MS, DHSc, RD, PA-C
Clinical Assistant Professor
Child Neurology and Pediatric Neurosurgery
Stanford University
Palo Alto, California

Ji ("CJ") Chun, PA-C, MPAS, BC-ADM
Endocrine Physician Assistant/Associate
OC Diabetes and Endocrinology
Fountain Valley, California
Adjunct Faculty
Physician Assistant Department
University of La Verne
La Verne, California
Past President
American Society of Endocrine PAs

Gregory L. Copeland, DO
Copeland Medical Healthcare Partners
Fresno, California

Gayani DeSilva, MD
Chief Physician, Psychiatry
LA DHS, Correctional Health
Child and Adolescent Psychiatrist
Inland Psychiatric Medical Group
Los Angeles, California

Milena Lopes Cavalcante, MD
Adventist Health
Fowler, California

Ariana O'Malley DMS, PA-C
Alumnus
Stanford University School of Medicine
Stanford, California

Alden Moir, MD
Ventura County Medical Center
Ventura, California

Sonia V. Otte, DMSc, MMS, PA-C
Founding Program Director
Associate Professor
Physician Assistant Program
California State University, San Bernardino
San Bernardino, California

Kristin Sato, DMS, PA-C
Physician Assistant
Department of Inpatient Hospital Medicine
Stanford Health Care
Stanford, California

Shannon Shieh, DMS, PA-C
Alumnus
Stanford University School of Medicine
Stanford, California

Benjamin Silverberg, MD, MSc, FAAFP, FCUCM
Associate Professor
Division of Ambulatory Operations, Department of Emergency Medicine
Medical Director
Division of Physician Assistant Studies
Department of Human Performance
West Virginia University School of Medicine
Morgantown, West Virginia

Greta Vines-Douglas, MSHS, PA-C
Program Director
School of Physician Assistant Studies
Marshall B. Ketchum University
Fullerton, California

Jennifer Weeks, DNP, FNP-C
Nurse Practitioner
MedNow
Evans, Georgia

Sampath Wijesinghe, DHSc, MS, MPAS, PA-C, AAHIVS
Clinical Associate Professor
Director of Career Development
Associate Director of Clerkship Education
MSPA Studies
Stanford School of Medicine
Primary Care PA-C and HIV Specialist
Copeland Medical Healthcare Partners
Clovis, California

Sahana Vishwanath MD, FACAAI
Allergy/Immunology
Adventist Health
Fowler, California

Reviewers of the Previous Edition

Krishan Ariyarathna, MD

Alan Brokenicky, MPAS, PA-C

Joan Caruso, MPAS, PA-C

Rachel Chappell, MHSc, PA-C

Simerjit Singh Dhaliwal, PA-C, MS, RCP

Christy Eskes, DHSc, MPA, PA-C

Michael Estrada, DHSc, MS, PA-C

Susan M. Fernandes, LPD, PA-C

Nichole A. Flores, BA, MA MAOB, PsyD

Jordan Hairr, EdD, MSPAS, PA-C

Virginia McCoy Hass, RN, DNP, FNP-C, PA-C

Megan Heidtbrink, MPAS, PA-C

Cherilyn M. Hendrix, DHEd, MSBME, PA-C, DFAAPA

Trenton Honda, PhD, MMS, PA-C

Amanda J. Ingalls, MS, PA-C

Jason R. Kessler, MD, FAAP

Rhonda Larsen, MHS, PA-C

Seth Lauterbach, MPAS, PA-C, CAQ-EM

Kevin Lohenry, PhD, PA-C

Stephanie McGilvray, PA-C, MMS

Jennifer Momen, MD, MPH, FAAP

Nina Multak, PhD, MPAS, PA-C, DFAAPA

Ila Naeni, DO

Ian Nelligan, MD, MPH

Courtney Nelson, MMS, PA-C

Jennifer Ramos, MPAP, PA-C

John Ramos, MMS, PA-C, EM-CAQ

Michele Toussaint, MS, PA-C

Judy Truscott, MPAS, PA-C

Joseph Weber, DHSc, MPAS, MBA, PA-C

Dee White, DNP, FNP

Sampath Wijesinghe, DHSc, MS, MPAS, PA-C, AAHIVS

Gordon H. Worley, MSN, RN, FNP-C, ENP-C

FOREWORD

I am thrilled to see this beautifully updated and revised edition of the outstanding book that Sampath Wijesinghe has created on primary care. The first edition of *101+ Primary Care Case Studies* has been a most valuable contribution, and the additions and modifications which have been made in the second edition make it even more valuable.

It is useful as a reference book for a specific case or problem, and it is also useful to learn about areas that may be unknown or a little known to the reader. I like to think of primary care as "whole person medicine" and certainly this book will help MDs, DOs, PAs, and nurse practitioners as a reference source as well as a primary guide.

Primary care continues to evolve as advances in medicine evolve. Thus, the need for a second edition which addresses these advances while building on a formidable base.

This is a remarkable collection of primary care case studies, presented in a unique and comprehensive manner. Included is a broad spectrum of cases that emphasize the scientific as well as the psychologic and emotional dimensions of care. We can all learn from each other as physicians, physician assistants, and nurse practitioners. Anyone interested in primary care will benefit from this book.

The book is arranged so you can pick and choose what interests you or relates to a specific case that you have. It is an ideal volume for those engaged in the primary care education of physicians, physician assistants, and nurse practitioners. It will also be a valuable resource for the primary care practitioner.

Besides the standard presentation of a patient problem, each case includes evidence-based information, references for additional reading, ICD-10 and CPT codes (very practical), topics for education, legal concerns, and specific items to be addressed by the broader healthcare team from receptionist to specialist. Bedside manner questions allow the educator or practitioner to expand the scope of inquiry, as time and interest permit. Finally, the narrative by the primary care provider brings the discussion from the didactic/scientific to the personal. I am not aware of any other volume that does this.

I congratulate Sampath Wijesinghe, who is a sterling example of a primary care educator and practitioner, for putting together this remarkable collection of cases and the stories that go with them. I know that the reader will find this multiauthored book invaluable and inspiring.

With great appreciation to Sam and his colleagues.

Alfred M. Sadler Jr., MD, FACP, ScD (Hon)
Senior Advisor
California State University
Master of Science Physician Assistant Program
Salinas, California

FOREWORD

Primary care medicine is the heart of medicine. It is a field where you never know what patient is going to walk through your door next. Frequently, what is listed on the schedule is not what you discover as you sit across from your patient and ask, "So what brings you in today?" It is also not what you discover when you dig a little deeper into a patient's story. More than once, I have called out to my puzzled medical assistant, "Can you grab me an anoscope?" for a patient who came in for a sore throat! Variety is part of what makes primary care so wonderful. As a clinician, you also get to build wonderful, long-term relationships, and this is my favorite part of primary care medicine. When you have seen patients year upon year, possibly even from birth, you really get to know them. In time, you recognize when there is a change in the way Mr. Jones is dressed, or note that his smile is a little less bright, or his steps a little more shuffled. There will likely be a day when your patient says "You saved my life" and rewards you with their homemade chocolates. There is never a dull day in primary care medicine, and as clinicians, we really make a difference in the population in which we serve. For these reasons, I love primary care medicine and there is no other place I would rather work as a nurse practitioner.

As a new clinician, you will really find it is true when that medicine is both art and science. You will develop your individual approach to the art of medicine. As you learn and grow, you will learn how to master your "medical paintbrush." You will see 10 clinicians might treat the same patient in 10 different ways, and all of them may be correct in their approaches. Listening carefully—*really listening*—to a patient, a family, and caregivers will improve your diagnostic skills. You will also learn how to most effectively and thoughtfully deliver education or bad news. Your clinical skills are absolutely vital, but your "soft skills" are invaluable. However, traditional classroom is not the most effective place to learn them. Soft skills come with time and experience and include communication skills, listening skills, and an ability to demonstrate empathy. It is your ability to "read" others. It is a vital part of our skill set as clinicians.

It is our job to earn our patients' trust and to give them the very best care. Even when our schedules are packed with back-to-back appointments and our inbox is stacked with labs and reports to be reviewed, we must remember that "the patient in Room 1" is more than just a CPT code. If primary care medicine is the heart of medicine, then our patients are its soul. We have to work collaboratively as a team—from the front office person, to the clinician, to the biller. We have to treat patients the way we would want to be treated because some day you may be the patient.

Clinical rotations can be an overwhelming experience for any student. Despite all of your didactic preparation, you may feel completely underprepared. The first year as a new clinician is a formidable learning trajectory. Suddenly, you are making life-and-death decisions about *your* patient. Apps and reference manuals are helpful, but what you really want is real-world advice from those in the trenches, and that is exactly what this book provides. It is a real-world, practical handbook of genuine scenarios. All the cases in the book are real-life case studies shared by the authors. Through a stepwise process, you will be challenged to critically think through the steps of clinical decision-making—from the chief complaint to billing and coding—they are all discussed. In addition to clinical decisions, you will hear each author's approach and some of the soft skills used. This book will be an invaluable asset, not only to a student or new clinician working in primary care but also to the seasoned professional who wants to gain insight by looking at other approaches in the art and science of medicine.

Lynn H. McComas, DNP, ANP-C, PHN
President/CEO PreceptorLink
Encinitas, California

FOREWORD

Some might say there are plenty of primary care textbooks today. Why one more? I am here to offer three reasons for *101+ Primary Care Case Studies*: the art, the appeal, and the author.

This text reminds us of the *art* of medicine, beyond the requirement to practice by evidence-based medicine. Yes, each case study provides the science and relevant practice guidelines behind a particular and vital diagnosis. To practice medicine solely by evidence alone leads to a risk of recipe-card decisions rather than personalized patient care. Heuristics, when conjoined with evidence, leads to best practice. *101+ Primary Care Case Studies* enhances this foundational evidence-based content, integrating the artistic touch of medicine by personalizing each case to a real patient. Each chapter includes the unique section, titled Insight From the PCP, which offers a clinician's pearls of wisdom about bedside manner and achieving optimal patient outcomes based on science and first-hand experience. The book's collection of pearls alone offers tremendous value to the reader seeking to guide patients toward the best health outcomes.

As it is written for primary care providers, this text emphasizes *the appeal* our career offers. In primary care, we have the privilege to develop patient relationships that extend across the lifespan. Representing these cradle-to-grave lives, the case studies in this book read as stories from the family. Only primary care expects a consistent patient relationship that celebrates births, school events, sporting achievements, graduations, marriages, promotions, relocations, retirements, and bereavements, with all the successes and disappointments along the journey. Clinical decisions wrestled in these pages are made with consideration of how it affects the individual life of a patient at a particular time. By reading only a handful of case studies herein, one comes away with how each patient deserves an individualized approach via team-based care with full consideration of the person's current life circumstances. That approach epitomizes why we in primary care love what we do.

Finally, to those who might say we have enough primary care textbooks, you do not know the author, Dr. Wijesinghe. He cares for his patients with both exceptional clinical skills and compassionate bedside manners, and emphasizes the importance of both to be a good clinician. He respects all members of the healthcare team as critical to optimal patient care, including receptionists, the cleaning crew, and the ever-important medical assistant. Dr. Wijesinghe seeks to be a part of the solution whenever possible (why he chose primary care medicine in rural clinics including HIV medicine, where healthcare professional shortages are the greatest). So, when using a textbook by an author with this indomitable spirit of integrity, the reader can expect an excellent opportunity to learn from a master among the most caring and professional of clinicians.

For learners entering the primary care professions of healthcare delivery, or for learners with years of medical experience, your library is incomplete without this book. Nothing else combines the art of medicine with the appeal of primary care better than what this author has created. We will serve our patients with better care by integrating the pearls of this text into our practices.

Michael J. Huckabee, PhD, MPAS, PA-C
Director, Physician Assistant Program
Associate Professor
Senior Associate Consultant-II
Mayo Clinic
Rochester, Minnesota

PREFACE

Introduction

Welcome to the second edition of *101+ Primary Care Case Studies*. When Springer Publishing approached me about the second edition of this book, I was deeply honored. The feedback I received during the first edition was truly heartening; many found the book instrumental in optimizing patient care. Some offered me invaluable insights to improve the second edition. To those who offered encouragement and praise, thank you for your ongoing support. And to those who provided constructive feedback, I listened attentively and integrated your suggestions into this new edition.

Medicine is a journey of lifelong learning, and the process of editing and authoring a book mirrors this pursuit. I continue to grow, drawing insights from fellow medical practitioners and educators, and staying current with advancements in medical knowledge. It is a privilege to be a perpetual student, and I am delighted to share what I learn with individuals like you.

I am confident that this second edition will serve both current and future clinicians, ultimately leading to improved patient outcomes.

Primary care medicine is the largest medical specialty in the United States. While physician associates, nurse practitioners, and physicians branch into specialties, a majority practices in primary care. When practicing primary care medicine, clinical skills and soft, or bedside manner, skills are important. Although there are many clinical medicine textbooks for students to learn all the important data about the hundreds of conditions a primary care provider will treat, there are few that use case studies as a primary means to help students work through a real patient scenario to strengthen clinical skills, let alone soft skills, which are often overlooked in a packed clinical curriculum. Current case study products typically focus solely on diagnostic skill. None focus on the combination of both clinical and bedside skills.

This book is intended to bridge the gap between the objective clinical content presented in the didactic phase of a PA, NP, or medical curriculum and the clinical application/rotation phase. It can be used during both phases of a program. Students will use book knowledge to work through a real-life chief complaint presented by a patient, and through a series of questions determine the appropriate focused exam, workup, diagnosis, and treatment for the patient.

Real-life medicine is not organized by organ system or diagnosis. Most often, patients will present with vague descriptions of symptoms, and a PCP will have to surmise the best approach to the problem. For example, a patient who presents with chest pain may have a diagnosis related to the heart, but the problem could also be related to anxiety or reflux.

The Origin of This Book

When I was a PA student, I enjoyed learning from clinicians who shared patient cases. I knew I would see similar cases when I started practice. When I began teaching at the University of California Davis PA/NP program, I taught students based on real cases. I recognized immediately that students are keen to learn from real cases. My experience first as a PA student and then as a medical educator led me to propose a book based on real cases. My initial idea was to write a book to help PA, NP, and medical students acquire competent skills.

Meeting Alex Moir

In August 2010, I started practicing primary care medicine in Sanger, a small town in California. I practiced medicine with Dr. Alex Moir, my collaborative physician. During my first week, Dr. Moir invited me to have lunch with him so we could get to know each other. I was looking forward to our lunch and was nervous at the same time. During our lunch, I said, “Dr. Moir, I am happy to work for you." He immediately corrected me, "Please don't think you work for me. I want you to know that you work *with* me. We are one team." On that day, I realized I had the opportunity to work with a great human being. Dr. Moir was my mentor, who practiced competent and compassionate care. I wanted to practice medicine like Dr. Moir practiced medicine. I always thought I was pretty compassionate, but, as I worked with Dr. Moir, I realized my compassionate care skills were developing even more. Dr. Moir was teaching me to deliver compassionate care. I was committed to sharing this powerful message with other clinicians, particularly with future clinicians, by keeping compassionate care central to the book's focus. So, I compiled this book based on real patient cases. I wanted Dr. Alex Moir to coauthor this book, but he died in a tragic accident. My grief put the book on hold for a time.

When I began to think about the book again, I decided I would dedicate it to Dr. Moir, whose mentorship influenced my life as a husband, father, and clinician. With that in mind, I reached out to some PCPs who provide competent and compassionate care to contribute cases. Some have taught me during my didactic training in PA school, some have trained me during my clinical clerkships, some are friends and colleagues, and some are students I had trained. I intentionally included a wide range of experience in this book, from very experienced clinicians to a few new clinicians. I wanted to present a variety of cases from clinicians with short-term and long-term experience. I hope these patient cases help future and practicing clinicians to learn and provide the best care to their patients. This book was a collaborative effort of many people with a common goal: taking care of patients and doing something meaningful for medical education.

The goal of this book is to improve competent skills and bedside skills. There is no disagreement that we can teach competence skills to the next generation and improve clinical skills. However, there is disagreement on whether compassion can be learned. I believe it can be, and there is evidence in support of my belief.

Compassion is fundamental to the delivery of healthcare,[1] something that patients, families, clinicians, and policy makers all agree.[2] The first principle of the American Medical Education cites compassion as being necessary in the delivery of care.[2] According to the Code of Ethics, "A physician shall be dedicated to providing competent medical care, with compassion and respect for human dignity and rights."[2] PAs and NPs are expected to practice the same. Consequently, compassion is required of all clinicians.

Are Bedside Skills and Compassion Practical to Teach?

There has been a long-term debate whether compassion can be taught. Some argue that compassion is an innate quality of character.[2] Current evidence suggests that compassion can be developed and sustained over time.[2] At the beginning of training, students demonstrate different levels of inherent compassion. Subsequently, capacity varies from student to student depending on their character at the baseline.[2] Recently, a randomized controlled trial on empathy training suggested that inherent qualities can be developed and sustained.[3]

Eight observational studies focused on educational interventions aimed at improving compassionate care provided by clinicians and students in a clinical setting.[4–12] The researchers used a variety methods (journals, simulations, reflection, etc.) and found that students demonstrate improved self-awareness, clinical communication skills, job satisfaction, caregiving competence, satisfaction with provision, and caregiver and workplace wellness.[4–12] Considering these results, it is safe to suggest that compassion is teachable.

Another group of authors found that common exemplary characteristics can improve humanistic behavior. Some of these were nonverbal communication, overt demonstrations of respect, building a personal connection, and eliciting and addressing patients' affective response to illness.[13] The authors concluded that there are many ways clinical teachers demonstrate humanistic behavior at the bedside.[13] Collectively, these findings suggest that as medical educators we have a role to play in teaching by example: Our humanistic behavior will build the same in students.[14] I am optimistic that the Insight From the PCP section of this book will reveal the art of medicine and be a valuable resource to promote a love of humanity.

Conclusion

Humanism and competent care are the primary focus of this book. If you are a PA, NP, or medical student, this will be a helpful and practical workbook during your education. These are real cases, so you know exactly what took place and how the cases were managed. To protect patients' privacy, names and other identifying information have been omitted, and some details about the cases were changed. Additionally, the authors who treated these patients do not have a byline on the case to further protect patient privacy. My goal is to share the practical aspect from each case and provide you an excellent learning opportunity while protecting every patient's privacy. Working through this book prior to clinical clerkships will provide a good foundation. Also, for practicing PCPs or clinicians about to enter practice, this book will be a helpful and practical resource.

When treating a patient, a PCP has an opportunity to provide comprehensive care that is both evidenced based and compassionate. All of us practicing clinicians and/or medical educators and future clinicians should be deliberate in our efforts to provide comprehensive care. It is my sincere hope that *101+ Primary Care Case Studies*, Second Edition, will continue to contribute to your ability to be a compassionate and competent PCP. Be well.

Sampath Wijesinghe

References

1. Sinclair S, Torres MB, Raffin-Bouchal S, et al. Compassion training in healthcare: what are patients' perspectives on training healthcare providers? *BMC Med Educ.* 2016;16:169. doi:10.1186/s12909-016-0695-0
2. Code of medical ethics. Principle 1. American Medical Association. 2001. https://code-medical-ethics.ama-assn.org/
3. Sinclair S, Norris JM, McConnell SJ, et al. Compassion: a scoping review of the healthcare literature. *BMC Palliat Care.* 2016;15:6. doi:10.1186/s12904-016-0080-0
4. Riess H, Kelley JM, Bailey RW, Dunn EJ, Phillips M. Empathy training for resident physicians: a randomized controlled trial of a neuroscience-informed curriculum. *J Gen Intern Med.* 2012;27(10):1280–1286. doi:10.1007/s11606-012-2063-z
5. Adamson E, Dewar B. Compassionate care: student nurses' learning through reflection and the use of story. *Nurse Educ Pract.* 2014;15(3):155–161. doi:10.1016/j.nepr.2014.08.002
6. Betcher DK. Elephant in the room project: improving caring efficacy through effective and compassionate communication with palliative care patients. *Medsurg Nurs.* 2010;19(2):101–105.
7. Blanco MA, Maderer A, Price LL, Epstein SK, Summergrad P. Efficiency is not enough; you have to prove that you care: role modelling of compassionate care in an innovative resident-as-teacher initiative. *Educ Health (Abingdon).* 2013;26(1):60–65. doi:10.4103/1357-6283.112805
8. Deloney LA, Graham CJ. Wit: using drama to teach first-year medical students about empathy and compassion. *Teach Learn Med.* 2003;15(4):247–251. doi:10.1207/s15328015tlm1504_06
9. Dewar B, Cook F. Developing compassion through a relationship centred appreciative leadership programme. *Nurse Educ Today.* 2014;34(9):1258–1264. doi:10.1016/j.nedt.2013.12.012
10. Fortney L, Luchterhand C, Zakletskaia L, Zgierska A, Rakel D. Abbreviated mindfulness intervention for job satisfaction, quality of life, and compassion in primary care clinicians: a pilot study. *Ann Fam Med.* 2013;11(5):412–420. doi:10.1370/afm.1511
11. Kalish R, Dawiskiba M, Sung YC, Blanco M. Raising medical student awareness of compassionate care through reflection of annotated videotapes of clinical encounters. *Educ Health (Abingdon).* 2011;24(3):490.
12. Shih CY, Hu WY, Lee LT, et al. Effect of a compassion-focused training program in palliative care education for medical students. *Am J Hosp Palliat Care.* 2013;30(2):114–120. doi:10.1177/1049909112445463
13. Weissmann PF, Branch WT, Gracey CF, Haidet P, Frankel RM. Role modeling humanistic behavior: learning bedside manner from the experts. *Acad Med J Assoc Am Med Coll.* 2006;81(7):661–667. doi:10.1097/01.ACM.0000232423.81299.fe
14. Institute of Medicine. *Improving Medical Education: Enhancing the Behavioral and Social Science Content of Medical School Curricula.* National Academies Press; 2004.

ACKNOWLEDGMENTS

I want to thank Springer Publishing Company for the opportunity to publish this book. Particularly, I would like to thank its executive acquisitions editor, Joseph Morita, and content development editor, Julia Curcio, for their support and guidance.

Second Edition

A total of six physicians, four NPs, and three PAs have contributed cases for this publication. Also, seven PAs, five physicians, and two NPs have served as peer reviewers. Thank you for your contributions and reviews.

First Edition

A total of 26 PAs, 12 NPs, and 13 physicians have contributed cases for this publication. Also, 25 PAs, 3 NPs, 5 physicians, and 1 psychologist have served as peer reviewers. Thank you for your contributions and reviews.

Time is priceless. As we age, we grow to understand the significance and value of each passing moment, especially the importance of cherishing time with loved ones. While I consistently prioritize spending time with my wife, Nuwan, and our children, Rynee and Ryler, there are moments when it becomes challenging due to my professional career. Your selflessness and unwavering support have been truly remarkable throughout my pursuits, including the publication of both the 1st and 2nd editions of this book. Your love and care mean the world to me, and I am grateful for your understanding and collaboration in our shared efforts to contribute, even in our small way, toward making the world a better place.

Dr. Ariana O'Malley, Dr. Kristin Sato, and Dr. Shannon Shieh for their expertise and editorial support. I am grateful for all your support!

HOW TO USE THIS BOOK

- Cases are organized by a patient's chief complaint, which is how a patient realistically presents in clinic.
- You will work through real-life patient cases* and answer a series of questions to determine the workup, diagnosis, and treatment for a patient. Except for question 6, the questions in each case are the same, to help guide you on how to methodically work through a patient's complaint. The questions are as follows:

1. **What is the differential diagnosis?** Pay careful attention to the history of present illness, review of systems, relevant history, and physical exam to determine a list of differential diagnoses. Provide a rationale for each diagnosis on your list. Briefly explain why or why not it is the most likely diagnosis.
2. **What is the most likely diagnosis? Why?** Based on the information available, determine the most likely diagnosis. Some cases are straightforward; others are not. That is the reality in primary care. Keep in mind you are making a most likely diagnosis, not a definitive diagnosis.
3. **Demonstrate your understanding about the pathophysiology of the most likely diagnosis.** While this is not a focus of the book, it is practical to have a basic understanding of a disease.
4. **Should tests/imaging studies be ordered? Which ones? Why? Think about tests/imaging beyond the primary care setting as well.** Determine what diagnostic testing and/or imaging is needed to evaluate the patient. What tests will be performed in the clinic? What tests or images might you want to order but are not typically available in a primary care setting? The online supplement provides details about the tests/imaging ordered by the PCP and other specialists involved in the case and also provides the results.
5. **What are the next appropriate steps in management?** Think about what your next steps would be for this patient. Are you going to treat and manage the patient? Would you transfer the patient to the ED? Would you refer to a specialist? If you are unclear how to move forward, check the online supplement to determine your progress and then move forward as appropriate.
6. **Review research on the diagnosis. Provide reference(s).** This question will vary from case to case, asking about risk factors, diagnostic criteria, prevalence, treatment options, and other information about the diagnosis under consideration. The use of evidence-based medicine is essential to stay abreast of recent developments, and no one has a greater need for an incredibly broad and deep knowledge base than a PCP. Read and rely on the best available research and refer to evidence whenever it is available. This, coupled with growing clinical expertise, is essential for practicing medicine. We are all lifelong learners.
7. **What are the pertinent ICD-10 and CPT (E/M) codes for this visit? Provide a short rationale.** ICD-10 has approximately 68,000 codes. Medical practitioners are expected to be specific when choosing these codes. This is an opportunity for future clinicians to learn how to do this. In addition, CPT (E/M) coding can be challenging for new clinicians.

*Demographics and patient data have been altered to protect privacy.

If there is an established patient with a medical diagnosis, clinicians may find it challenging to determine whether the visit is coded as level 3 or level 4. This exercise builds this skill. In the second edition of the book, we have introduced time-based billing, a widely adopted method among primary care providers today.

8. **What is the appropriate patient education topic for this case?** PCPs have a responsibility to educate patients on disease, diagnosis, treatment, and good health habits. This is mandatory and part of every patient visit.
9. **If not managed appropriately, what is/are the medical/legal concern(s) that may arise?** Despite training and experience, there are rare occasions when a negative patient outcome or experience leads to legal action or medical consequence. It is important that young clinicians identify areas of legal exposure and the consequences of incorrect diagnoses and negligence.
10. **Think about interprofessional collaboration for this case. Provide a list of specialties or other disciplines and indicate what contribution these professionals might make to managing the patient.** Medicine is a team sport. PCPs cannot do their jobs alone. It is essential that clinicians value each team member and recognize their contributions. This question will help you become aware of how many individuals actually contribute to a patient's care.

- The cases conclude with a question or questions about your personal bedside manner approach, including communication, handling a distressed patient or parent, and dealing with negative outcomes. These are subjective questions for which answers are not directly provided but are intended to be thought provoking and to encourage discussion.
- Pay careful attention to the history of present illness, review of systems, relevant history, and physical exam to determine the best answers to these questions.
- Answers to all the questions are available on Springer Publishing CourseConnect. Instructions for how to access CourseConnect appear on the CourseConnect access card that accompanies this book. Try to answer the questions yourself before reviewing the answers and outcomes online.
- Note that the answers for the bedside manner questions are somewhat subjective. The Outcome and Insight From the PCP sections available online demonstrate the author's bedside manner and compassion and how the case developed and concluded. The insights from the PCPs provide valuable information about effective communication skills and ways to build trust and underscore the importance of a PCP–patient relationship.
- Keep in mind that medicine is subjective, and clinicians have different approaches to managing patients. They may come up with the same diagnosis at the end; however, their approaches will likely differ.
- For instructors who are using this workbook in a classroom environment, a filterable table of contents is available to you to sort through cases by diagnosis, patient population, gender, and organ system to aid in assignments. Contact your Springer Publishing sales representative for access at springerpub.com/instructors.
- A breakdown of the number of cases by system appears below (*Note:* This count includes the online cases available for instructors. Some cases belong to two systems.):
  - Behavioral Medicine 8
  - Cardiovascular System 9
  - Dermatologic System 5
  - Endocrine System 8
  - Eyes, Ears, Nose, and Throat 10
  - Gastrointestinal System 13
  - Genitourinary System 10
  - Hematology/Oncology 8
  - Infectious Disease/Reproductive System 4
  - Infectious Disease 15
  - Musculoskeletal System 15
  - Neurologic System 9
  - Pulmonary System 10
  - Renal System 4
  - Reproductive System 6

INSTRUCTOR RESOURCES

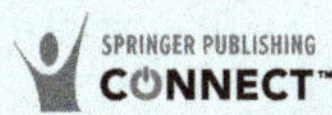

A robust set of instructor resources designed to supplement this text is located at **http://connect.springerpub.com/content/book/978-0-8261-3968-9.** Qualifying instructors may request access by emailing **textbook@springerpub.com.**

- LMS Common Cartridge—All Instructor Resources
- Online-Only Cases—25 Additional Case Studies
- Instructor Table of Contents, Filterable by Body System and Population

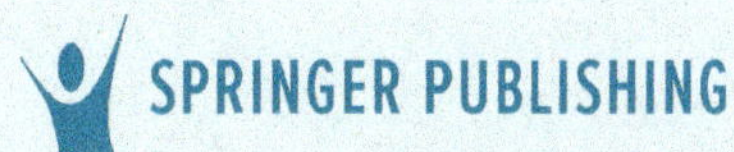

Visit https://connect.springerpub.com/ and look for the "**Show Supplementary**" button on the book **homepage**.

PART I: ADULT

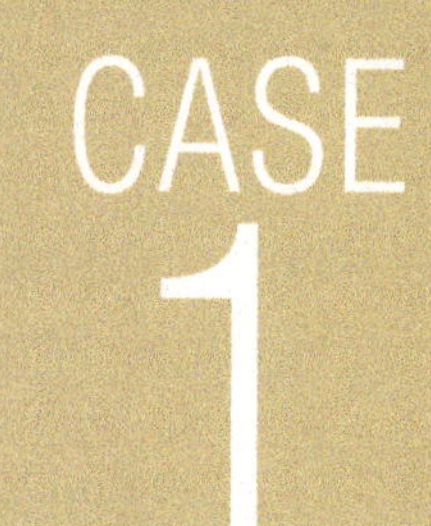

DYSPNEA AND RIGHT-SIDE CHEST PAIN, ADULT MALE

Chief Complaint

"Shortness of breath, pain in the right side of chest."

History of Present Illness

A 23-year-old male presents to the PCP with sudden onset of right-sided chest pain and transient SOB while lifting a box onto a moving truck. Patient states he felt sudden pain while at work as a mover. He denies any trauma, recent illness, travel, or sick contacts. Associated with the pain was a brief episode of difficulty breathing. He states the pain is worsened by lifting his right arm or standing up straight.

The patient reports he was loading boxes onto a moving truck. He lifted a box overhead and felt a sudden "pull" and sharp pain to the upper right side of his anterior chest wall. This was associated with a transient period of SOB. The breathing resolved as soon as he put the box down, lowered his arm, and leaned forward. Pain worsens if he tries to stand up straight or lift his right arm. Pain improves if he leans forward.

He lives at home with his parents who are alive and well. He works full time as mover/laborer, drinks two to four alcoholic beverages per week, and has smoked half a pack of cigarettes daily for 5 years. Patient denies any recent illness, fever, chills, constitutional symptoms, weight loss, cough, congestion, or sick contacts.

Review of Systems

ROS is significant for a brief episode of difficulty breathing associated with pain to the right side of his chest. ROS is negative for any breaks in the skin, rashes, or bites. The patient denies any recent domestic or international travel. He denies any new CNS, heart, GI, and GU symptoms.

Relevant History

The patient reports being healthy and having no significant medical issues nor surgeries. He states he had routine wellness visits and his immunizations are up to date.

Allergies

No known drug allergies; no known food allergies.

Medications

None.

Physical Examination

- *Vitals:* T 37.1°C (98.7°F), P 66, R 16, BP 120/78, SpO_2 98%, HT 198 cm (78 in.), WT 74.8 kg (165 lb), BMI 19.1.
- *General:* Well-appearing, tall, lean 23-year-old male in no acute distress, standing leaning forward with left hand on right upper chest below the clavicle.
- *Psychiatric:* Affect and mood are appropriate to setting.
- *Skin, Hair, and Nails:* No rashes, no burns noted, brisk capillary refill in both hands.
- *Head:* No evidence of trauma, bleeding, or bruising.

- *ENT/Mouth:* Trachea midline.
- *Neck:* Supple, no lymphadenopathy noted.
- *Chest:* Symmetric, no pain with palpation, no palpable deformity.
- *Lungs:* Diminished lung sounds in the right upper chest, otherwise clear to auscultation in remaining fields.
- *Heart:* Regular rate and rhythm, no murmurs noted on auscultation.
- *Abdomen:* Soft, nontender, no guarding or rebound.
- *Genital/Rectal:* Deferred.
- *Musculoskeletal:* No gross deformities noted to spine, chest wall, and upper or lower extremities.
- *Neurologic:* Walks leaning forward and to the right with left hand on right upper chest. Strength equal and intact in upper and lower extremities.
- *Vascular:* Skin is warm to touch; pulses are equal and intact in the upper and lower extremities.

Clinical Discussion Questions

1. What is the differential diagnosis?

2. What is the most likely diagnosis? Why?

3. Demonstrate your understanding about the pathophysiology of the most likely diagnosis.

4. Should tests/imaging studies be ordered? Which ones? Why? Think about tests/imaging beyond the primary care setting as well.

5. What are the next appropriate steps in management?

6. How does this medical condition in a child adversely affect an entire family? Provide references for your response.

7. What are the pertinent ICD-10 and CPT (E/M) codes for this visit? Provide a short rationale.

8. What is the appropriate patient education topic for this case?

9. If not managed appropriately, what is/are the medical/legal concern(s) that may arise?

10. Think about interprofessional collaboration for this case. Provide a list of specialties or other disciplines and indicate what contribution these professionals might make to managing the patient.

BEDSIDE MANNER QUESTION

11. What would your communication style/approach be with this patient?

Answers available at courseconnect.springerpub.com.

CASE 2

FATIGUE AND WEAKNESS, ADULT FEMALE

Chief Complaint

"Fatigue and weakness."

History of Present Illness

A 52-year-old White woman presents to her PCP with complaints of increasing fatigue and weakness over the past 3 to 4 months. She is an avid runner and finds it difficult to keep her usual distance or pace. She tried adding a multivitamin to her daily regimen and has been tracking her sleep on an exercise-tracking watch for the past month without significant findings. She does report having some irregularity with her menses over this past year, but her routine gynecologic exam showed no significant concerns and she denies excessive or heavy bleeding. Her gynecologist reportedly told her she is likely in perimenopause after confirming she is not pregnant with an in-office urine hCG, and she has a follow-up appointment scheduled in about 6 weeks. The patient denies any anxiety or depression and reports good social activity. Her diet is vegetarian and reported to be well balanced.

Review of Systems

The patient's ROS is positive for asthenia without anorexia or weight loss and positive for angular cheilosis and increased soreness of tongue and mouth at times, and she does note some mild hair loss and brittle nails. Her ROS is also positive for some dyspnea on exertion and exercise intolerance, and she has some constipation. She denies chest pain or palpitations. The ROS is also negative for abdominal pain, nausea, vomiting, or diarrhea. She denies blood in stools, hematuria, or dysuria. The patient also denies dizziness, blurred vision, headache, anxiety, and depression. She denies fever, chills, and night sweats and has had no significant change in weight or unusual bruising reported.

Relevant History

The patient's history is unremarkable. Her menses are irregular, less frequent for the past 9 months, with her last menstrual period about 8 weeks ago without excessive or heavy bleeding. Her surgical history is significant for one cesarean section at age 28 and appendectomy at age 35.

The patient is married and lives at home with her spouse and youngest child. She is employed as an accountant full time with a graduate school education. She denies smoking or illicit drug use. She drinks socially, reporting about four to five glasses of wine per week. Her family history includes her mother, aged 76, with hypertension, and father, aged 77, with hyperlipidemia, hypertension, and gout.

Allergies

Fluoroquinolones (rash); no known food allergies.

Medications

- Women's over-50 multivitamin.
- Occasional ibuprofen 400 mg PRN for pain.

PHYSICAL EXAMINATION

- *Vitals:* T 36°C (96.8°F), P 62, R 14, BP 112/62, HT 170 cm (67 in.), WT 57 kg (126 lb), BMI 19.4.
- *General:* A&O×3, well groomed.
- *Psychiatric:* Normal affect, pleasant and cooperative.
- *Skin, Hair, and Nails:* Skin dry but without rash or lesions, normal hair distribution, brittle nails.
- *Eye:* Mild pallor of the conjunctiva.
- *ENT/Mouth:* Evidence of healing angular cheilosis bilaterally with some smoothness and redness of the tongue. Mucous membranes with some mild pallor.
- *Neck:* Supple without thyromegaly. Head and neck lymph nodes within normal limits.
- *Lungs:* Clear to auscultation with normal respiratory effort.
- *Heart:* S1S2, RRR; no murmur noted.
- *Abdomen:* Soft, nontender, no distention. No organomegaly. Positive and normal bowel sounds in all quadrants.
- *Genital/Rectal:* No external hemorrhoids, negative for occult blood. Genital exam deferred.
- *Neurologic:* CN II–XII grossly intact with normal patellar deep tendon reflexes.

CLINICAL DISCUSSION QUESTIONS

1. What is the differential diagnosis?

2. What is the most likely diagnosis? Why?

3. Demonstrate your understanding about the pathophysiology of the most likely diagnosis.

4. Should tests/imaging studies be ordered? Which ones? Why? Think about tests/imaging beyond the primary care setting as well.

5. What are the next appropriate steps in management?

6. What are the causes, risk factors, and treatment options for this diagnosis? Provide references for your response.

7. What are the pertinent ICD-10 and CPT (E/M) codes for this visit? Provide a short rationale.

8. What is the appropriate patient education topic for this case?

9. If not managed appropriately, what is/are the medical/legal concern(s) that may arise?

10. Think about interprofessional collaboration for this case. Provide a list of specialties or other disciplines and indicate what contribution these professionals might make to managing the patient.

Bedside Manner Questions

11. How would you communicate your likely diagnosis to the patient?

12. If the patient shows distress at what you communicate, how would you provide support?

Answers available at courseconnect.springerpub.com.

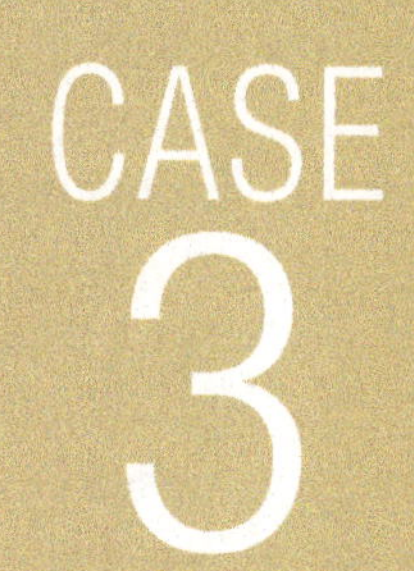

LEFT HIP PAIN, ADULT FEMALE

CASE 3

Chief Complaint

"Left hip pain."

History of Present Illness

A 55-year-old woman presents with an ongoing complaint of left hip pain. She had been doing physical therapy as ordered and is back to the office to learn her x-ray results.

Her initial injury was approximately 2 months prior when she had come in with concern about an inguinal/groin strain. She was working full time as an MA for a local home health agency. On the day of the injury, she heard a pop in her left hip while transferring an older adult patient. Her groin felt tight, "like a vise around my pelvis," but she was able to continue working for another 6 weeks. She came to the clinic initially with a request for physical therapy. She was also started on ibuprofen 600 mg by mouth, three times a day.

She returned to the clinic after 3 weeks and saw a different provider. Her PT shifted emphasis from her groin to her left hip, but this did not help, and she reported that "the pain was worse" following exercise. The provider prescribed low-dose narcotics and a muscle relaxant. A left hip x-ray was ordered, as well as a pelvic ultrasound and x-ray of the lumbar spine.

The patient then sent the PCP an electronic message through her EHR requesting short-term disability because she did not feel safe lifting or transferring bed-bound patients.

Prior to her injury, she had been going to the gym three times per week to lift weights but denies any activity that may have hurt her hip in the past. She was a long-distance runner 5 years ago but stopped because of time constraints. She is single, has two adult children, and is normally healthy.

Her last laboratory tests, performed 3 months before injury, were in the normal range.

Review of Systems

The patient's ROS is positive for left hip pain with active ROM and constipation when using narcotics. The ROS is negative for limping, numbness, or tingling in the left foot, and she has no back pain.

Relevant History

Her medical history is significant for childhood asthma (unknown treatment), trigger finger and arthritis in left thumb (age 48), heartburn (age 50), varicose veins in the bilateral lower extremities (age 52), and pain in both feet (age 54). Her surgical history includes a tubal ligation and a right thumb trigger release. The patient was a previous smoker (23 pack years) but quit 12 years ago. She rarely drinks alcohol and uses no recreational drugs. She has not been sexually active for "a couple of years." She lives alone, exercises regularly, and has two grown children. Her family history is positive for mesothelioma (deceased father), obesity, type 2 diabetes (deceased mother), and lung cancer (deceased grandfather).

Allergies

Erythromycin (stomach upset).

Medications

Ibuprofen 600 mg PO TID PRN pain.

PHYSICAL EXAMINATION

- *Vitals:* T 36.4°C (97.6°F), P 78, R 16, BP 116/72, HT 172.5 cm (68 in.), WT 72.6 kg (160 lb), SpO_2 99% (room air), BMI 24.14.
- *General:* Well-appearing female, mild discomfort with movement in and out of sitting position. Appears stated age.
- *Psychiatric:* Mildly anxious.
- *Skin, Hair, and Nails:* Skin normal in appearance, no rashes or lesions. Normal hair distribution. Nail beds pink with no cyanosis/clubbing.
- *Head:* Normal shape and appearance.
- *Eyes:* Conjunctivae are clear without exudates or hemorrhage. Sclera is nonicteric. Bilateral. Extraocular muscle intact; pupils equal, round, and reactive to light and accommodation. Eyelids are normal in appearance without swelling or lesions.
- *ENT/Mouth:* The external ears are nontender and without swelling; hearing grossly intact. Nose has no obstruction or discharge. Oropharynx has no inflammation, swelling, exudate, or lesion. Mouth with no lesions; dentition good.
- *Neck:* Supple with no adenopathy.
- *Lungs:* Lung sounds clear in all lobes.
- *Heart:* Rate and rhythm are normal.
- *Abdomen:* Soft, nontender, no masses or guarding.
- *Musculoskeletal:* Leg length equal; sacroiliac stress tests positive for three of five tests: distraction, no pain; thigh thrust, no pain; FABER, positive for pain. Compression, positive for pain. Gaenslen's maneuver, positive for pain. Gait without limp.
- *Neurologic:* A&O to person/place/time, color/sensation/movement within normal limits on bilateral legs and feet.

CLINICAL DISCUSSION QUESTIONS

1. What is the differential diagnosis?

___

___

___

___

2. What is the most likely diagnosis? Why?

___

___

___

___

3. Demonstrate your understanding about the pathophysiology of the most likely diagnosis.

___

___

___

___

4. Should tests/imaging studies be ordered? Which ones? Why? Think about tests/imaging beyond the primary care setting as well.

5. What are the next appropriate steps in management?

6. What are the risk factors, causes, and most common site for this diagnosis? Provide references for your response.

7. What are the pertinent ICD-10 and CPT (E/M) codes for this visit? Provide a short rationale.

8. What is the appropriate patient education topic for this case?

9. If not managed appropriately, what is/are the medical/legal concern(s) that may arise?

10. Think about interprofessional collaboration for this case. Provide a list of specialties or other disciplines and indicate what contribution these professionals might make to managing the patient.

Bedside Manner Questions

11. How would you communicate your likely diagnosis to the patient?

12. If the patient shows distress at what you communicate, how would you provide support?

13. If diagnostic evidence points to a more complicated case that could potentially result in a negative outcome, how would you communicate this possibility?

Answers available at courseconnect.springerpub.com.

CASE 4

VAGINAL BLEEDING, ADULT FEMALE

Chief Complaint

"Vaginal bleeding."

History of Present Illness

A 28-year-old woman presents to her PCP with a 3-day history of dizziness, fatigue, and headache. She is the mother of two girls, ages 5 and 2. She and her husband want another child, have planned accordingly, and are hoping for a boy. She missed her last period and suspects she is pregnant; a home pregnancy test taken last week was positive. Until 3 days ago, she felt fine, other than some fatigue and mild nausea. Over the last 2 days, she began experiencing abdominal cramping and irregular vaginal bleeding. She points to both lower and upper quadrants as the main location of the pain. She describes her abdominal pain as 7 out of 10. She has not used over-the-counter pain medication because she wants to avoid medication if pregnant. Additionally, she states, "When changing positions, I get lightheaded." When the PCP asks about her bleeding, she states she has had similar bleeding during her other pregnancies. "All my pregnancies are like that. It's normal."

Review of Systems

The ROS is positive for fatigue, nausea, abdominal pain, and vaginal bleeding. The patient reports headache and dizziness. The ROS is negative for fever, chills, vomiting, diarrhea, constipation, SOB, or chest pain.

Relevant History

The patient's medical history is significant for cholecystectomy (age 27) and chlamydia infection (age 17). Her social history includes drinking one glass of wine per weekend since age 18. She had a few male sex partners prior to her marriage. She lives with her husband and children and describes her marriage as happy. Both children were full-term babies and the pregnancies were normal. Her family history is unknown as she was adopted.

Allergies

No known drug allergies; no known food allergies.

Medications

None.

Physical Examination

- *Vitals:* T 37°C (98.6°F), P 70, R 19, BP 130/80, WT 78.7 kg (173.5 lb), HT 167.6 cm (66 in.), BMI 28.
- *General:* Appears anxious and fatigued, mild acute distress.
- *Skin, Hair, and Nails:* No rash, skin warm and dry. No abnormal findings with hair or nails.
- *Lungs:* Clear to auscultation bilaterally, good air movement throughout.
- *Heart:* RRR, without murmur or gallop.
- *Abdomen:* Abdomen was soft, nondistended, and moderately tender; generalized.
- *Neurologic:* A&O×3, cranial nerves II to XII grossly intact.

CLINICAL DISCUSSION QUESTIONS

1. What is the differential diagnosis?

2. What is the most likely diagnosis? Why?

3. Demonstrate your understanding about the pathophysiology of the most likely diagnosis.

4. Should tests/imaging studies be ordered? Which ones? Why? Think about tests/imaging beyond the primary care setting as well.

5. What are the next appropriate steps in management?

6. Demonstrate your understanding about the most common location of the diagnosis, risk factors, and treatment options. Provide reference for your responses.

7. What are the pertinent ICD-10 and CPT (E/M) codes for this visit? Provide a short rationale.

8. What is the appropriate patient education topic for this case?

9. If not managed appropriately, what is/are the medical/legal concern(s) that may arise?

10. Think about interprofessional collaboration for this case. Provide a list of specialties or other disciplines and indicate what contribution these professionals might make to managing the patient.

BEDSIDE MANNER QUESTIONS

11. What would your communication style/approach be with this patient?

12. If a patient is distressed by the diagnosis, what might offer support?

Answers available at courseconnect.springerpub.com.

CASE 5

FEVER AND BODY ACHES, ADULT MALE

Chief Complaint

"Fever and body aches."

History of Present Illness

A 27-year-old man presents to his PCP with a history of fever, chills, sore throat, body aches, and headache. He states, "I have been having fevers, chills, fatigue, sore throat, body aches, and headache for the last 4 days. I thought I would be better by now, but I think I am getting worse. I just returned from a vacation in Papua New Guinea. I think I have the seasonal flu or malaria. I did not have a chance to get this year's flu shot or malaria prevention medicine prior to my trip. I need your help, please." The patient is a music teacher who loves traveling with a group every winter. About 4 weeks ago, he went on a vacation to tropical New Guinea. He admits to having unprotected sex with a woman in the travel group as well as unprotected sex with a local man. He is concerned because his symptoms are not improving. He has been resting and drinking plenty of fluids. In addition, he has been taking ibuprofen 400 mg every 6 hours PRN for his fever. Ibuprofen has reduced his fever slightly and helped him with his body aches, sore throat, and headache. As the patient states, his fever has been consistent and the only way he can manage it is by taking ibuprofen. He states, "I have some family members with flu-like symptoms and met them for a short time last week during a family event." He denies any other symptoms.

Review of Systems

The patient is positive for fevers, chills, sore throat, and body aches. He reports fatigue and headache. The ROS is negative for diarrhea, constipation, nausea, vomiting, rash, runny nose, cough, urinary urgency, dysuria, back pain, abdominal pain, penile discharge, night sweat, diaphoresis, loss of appetite, SOB, or chest pain.

Relevant History

The patient's medical history is significant for an appendectomy (age 15) and gonorrhea (age 23). He has no chronic medical problems. Currently, he is not taking any medication other than ibuprofen. His social history includes drinking eight beers over the weekend. He has had three female sex partners and one male partner during the last year. His family history includes a father with benign prostatic hyperplasia, hypertension, and T2DM and a mother with T2DM and breast cancer. His siblings (two sisters and one brother) are younger, and their medical histories are unremarkable.

Allergies

No known drug allergies; no known food allergies.

Medications

Ibuprofen 400 mg every 6 hours PRN.

Physical Examination

- *Vitals:* T 39.4°C (102.9°F), P 84, R 18, BP 140/89, WT 71.7 kg (158 lb), HT 172.7 cm (68 in.), BMI 24.
- *General:* Febrile; appears anxious and fatigued; NAD.
- *Psychiatric:* Cooperative; appropriate mood and affect.

- *Skin, Hair, and Nails:* No skin rash or lesions. No abnormal findings with hair and nail exam.
- *Eyes:* Conjunctiva and sclera clear.
- *ENT/Mouth:* In normal limits, except for mild rhinorrhea.
- *Neck:* Bilateral anterior cervical lymphadenopathy; no posterior cervical lymph nodes.
- *Lungs:* Clear with good air movement.
- *Heart:* RRR; no murmur or gallop.
- *Abdomen:* Soft, nontender, not distended; no organomegaly.
- *Neurologic:* A&O×3.

Clinical Discussion Questions

1. What is the differential diagnosis?

2. What is the most likely diagnosis? Why?

3. Demonstrate your understanding about the pathophysiology of the most likely diagnosis.

4. Should tests/imaging studies be ordered? Which ones? Why? Think about tests/imaging beyond the primary care setting as well.

5. What are the next appropriate steps in management?

6. Review recent and credible research article(s) on this diagnosis. Demonstrate your understanding about the transmission, screening tests, and treatment initiation. Provide references for your response(s).

7. What are the pertinent ICD-10 and CPT (E/M) codes for this visit? Provide a short rationale.

8. What is the appropriate patient education topic for this case?

9. If not managed appropriately, what is/are the medical/legal concern(s) that may arise?

10. Think about interprofessional collaboration for this case. Provide a list of specialties or other disciplines and indicate what contribution these professionals might make to managing the patient.

BEDSIDE MANNER QUESTIONS

11. What would your communication style/approach be with this patient?

12. If a patient is distressed by the diagnosis, what might offer support?

Answers available at courseconnect.springerpub.com.

CASE 6

BLURRY VISION, ADULT FEMALE

Chief Complaint

"Blurry vision."

History of Present Illness

A 32-year-old otherwise healthy woman presents to her PCP complaining of blurred vision; light headedness; diplopia; and numbness in her lower extremities, tongue, and left side of her face. The symptoms became increasingly worse; over a period of 2 months and then began to improve with complete resolution of symptoms by the fourth month. The patient reported no relieving or aggravating factors while the symptoms were present.

Review of Systems

The ROS is positive for rash to the anterior chest; occasional headache; double vision; blurred vision; numbness in the lower extremities, tongue, and left side of the face; and anxiety related to current symptoms. The ROS is negative for weight change, hearing loss, tinnitus, epistaxis, SOB, chest pain, cough, nausea, vomiting, diarrhea, abdominal pain, urinary symptoms, bruising, or temperature intolerance.

Relevant History

The patient's medical history is significant for measles at the age of 9 months and infectious mononucleosis at the age of 20. She wears glasses and contacts. Her family history is significant for HTN in both her mother and father; her maternal grandfather has chronic renal failure. Her social history includes a 15-pack-year history of tobacco use, no alcohol, and no illicit drug use. She lives with her husband and their golden retriever.

Allergies

No known drug allergies; no known food allergies.

Medications

None.

Physical Examination

- *Vitals:* T 37.2°C (99.0°F), P 92, R 16, BP 122/72, WT 61.70 kg (136 lb), HT 167.64 cm (66 in.), BMI 22.
- *General:* Healthy appearing, well-dressed, well-groomed female in no apparent distress.
- *Skin, Hair, and Nails:* Small and erythematous papules on the anterior chest under bilateral breasts. No abnormal findings with hair or nails.
- *Head:* Atraumatic, normocephalic.
- *Eyes:* EOM reveals a sixth nerve palsy of the left eye, decreased visual acuity of the right eye (OD 20/40) with an enlarged cup-to-disc ratio; PERRL.
- *Lungs:* CTA bilaterally.
- *Heart:* RRR; no murmurs, rubs, or gallops.
- *Lymphatic:* No lymphadenopathy noted.

- *Neurologic:* Positive Lhermitte sign; decreased sensation from L2 to L5 and S1 of the lower extremities; DTR of bilateral lower extremities 1+ with decreased sensation of the tongue and of the ophthalmic nerve distribution of the left side of the face.

CLINICAL DISCUSSION QUESTIONS

1. What is the differential diagnosis?

2. What is the most likely diagnosis? Why?

3. Demonstrate your understanding of the pathophysiology of the most likely diagnosis.

4. Should tests/imaging studies be ordered? Which ones? Why? Think about tests/imaging beyond the primary care setting as well.

5. What are the next appropriate steps in management?

6. Review a recent and credible research article(s) about this diagnosis. Demonstrate your understanding of the diagnostic criteria, risk factors, and treatment options. Include a list of your reference(s).

7. What are the pertinent ICD-10 and CPT (E/M) codes for this visit? Provide a short rationale.

8. What is the appropriate patient education topic for this case?

9. If not managed appropriately, what is/are the medical/legal concern(s) that may arise?

10. Think about interprofessional collaboration for this case. Provide a list of specialties or other disciplines and indicate what contribution these professionals might make to managing the patient.

BEDSIDE MANNER QUESTIONS

11. What would your communication style/approach be with this patient?

12. If a patient is distressed by the diagnosis, what might offer support?

____

____

____

____

Answers available at courseconnect.springerpub.com.

CASE 7

FREQUENT URINATION, ADULT MALE

Chief Complaint

"Frequent urination."

History of Present Illness

A 42-year-old man with a history of HTN and substance use disorder comes to the primary care clinic for a mandatory health checkup. He is on court probation and living in a sober house that requires an intake physical exam. He complains of fatigue, frequent urination, excessive thirst, and blurred vision. He also reports gradual weight gain and tingling and numbness in his extremities, which make performing chores in the sober house difficult. His symptoms started about 2 years ago but have never been checked as he has been in and out of jail. His urination frequency and the volume output are getting worse. He reports seeing ants around the toilet bowl every morning for about 2 weeks. He drinks a lot of water (about half a gallon daily), but there has been no improvement. He was concerned about these symptoms because his older brother was diagnosed with DM and both parents had died from complications of DM. In the past, he used cocaine to relax and not worry about his symptoms.

Review of Systems

The ROS is positive for symptoms related to the HPI: polyuria, polydipsia, paresthesia, blurred vision, fatigue, and weight gain. The patient reports dry skin, cuts, and bruises that are slow to heal; poor dentition; and abdominal bloating. He reports cravings and feeling down but denies significant opioid withdrawal symptoms. The ROS is negative for fever, chills, headaches, diarrhea, or vomiting. He denies any blood in the urine, dysuria, or urge incontinence and has no known history of STDs. He has no chest pain, stomachache, backache, extremity pain, or edema.

Relevant History

The patient has a medical history of HTN (diagnosed 5 years prior but is not on antihypertensives when he comes to the clinic). He also has a history of substance use disorder involving inhaled cocaine and occasional IV heroin use. He had recently seen a behavioral health specialist at the sober house. He has no history of surgery or hospitalization. Both parents died in their early 60s from complications of DM. An older brother was diagnosed with T2DM at age 42 and prostate cancer at age 50. His younger sister is in good health. Since graduating from high school, he has worked as a truck driver, transporting alcoholic beverages from Connecticut to Florida. He is planning to resume this job after completing his court probation. He is divorced and has two adult sons; both are in good health. For a long time, he depended on fast foods and never had time to exercise. He uses alcohol socially and smokes half a pack of cigarettes per day. He is unemployed and uninsured and has no support system except for the counselors at the sober house.

Allergies

No known drug allergies; no known food allergies.

Medications

Methadone (50 mg daily); directly observed therapy at the methadone clinic.

PHYSICAL EXAMINATION

- *Vitals:* T 37°C (98.6°F), P 80, R 14, BP 150/88, WT 109 kg (240.3 lb), HT 175 cm (68.9 in.), waist circumference 42 in., BMI 35.6.
- *General:* Well-developed and well-nourished middle-aged African American man in no acute distress.
- *Psychiatric:* Mildly anxious with a flat affect.
- *Skin, Hair, and Nails:* Skin dry with discoloration in body folds, no rashes or bleeding tendency. Hair intact. Nails yellow and brittle.
- *Head:* Normocephalic.
- *Eyes:* Vision reduced bilaterally; PERRL. Intraretinal hemorrhages, exudates, and cotton wool spots in both eyes.
- *ENT/Mouth:* TM pearly, grey with no fluid. Oral mucosa moist; dentition in bad repair with easy gum bleeding.
- *Neck:* Supple with no adenopathy or thyroid enlargement.
- *Chest:* No deformities noted.
- *Lungs:* CTA bilaterally.
- *Breasts:* Nontender; no lumps.
- *Heart:* RRR, without murmurs, gallops, or rubs.
- *Peripheral Vascular:* Faint dorsalis pedis and posterior tibial pulses (1/4).
- *Abdomen:* Soft with no masses, organomegaly, or tenderness. Active bowel sounds in all four quadrants.
- *Genital/Rectal:* No penile or testicular abnormalities noted. Prostate within normal limits.
- *Lymphatics:* No axillary or inguinal lymphadenopathy.
- *Musculoskeletal:* No deformities, tenderness, or edema. FROM in all joints.
- *Neurologic:* A&O×3; cranial nerves II to XII grossly intact. Reflexes present in all extremities. Mild defects on proprioception, vibration, and monofilament sensation.
- *Point-of-Care Testing:* Point-of-care laboratory testing revealed a random BG of 340 mg/dL, 3+ glucose in urine, and no ketones. Hgb A1C was 8.8%.

CLINICAL DISCUSSION QUESTIONS

1. What is the differential diagnosis?

____

____

____

____

____

2. What is the most likely diagnosis? Why?

____

____

____

____

3. Demonstrate your understanding about the pathophysiology of the most likely diagnosis.

4. Should tests/imaging studies be ordered? Which ones? Why? Think about tests/imaging beyond the primary care setting as well.

5. What are the next appropriate steps in management?

6. Review a recent and credible research article(s) about this diagnosis. Demonstrate your understanding of the prevalence, diagnostic criteria, and treatment options. Include a list of reference(s).

7. What are the pertinent ICD-10 and CPT (E/M) codes for this visit? Provide a short rationale.

8. What are the appropriate patient education topics for this case?

9. If not managed appropriately, what is/are the medical/legal concern(s) that may arise?

10. Think about interprofessional collaboration for this case. Provide a list of specialties or other disciplines and indicate what contribution these professionals might make to managing the patient.

Bedside Manner Questions

11. What would your communication style/approach be with this patient?

12. If a patient is distressed by the diagnosis, what might offer support?

Answers available at courseconnect.springerpub.com.

MEDICATION ADJUSTMENT, ADULT MALE

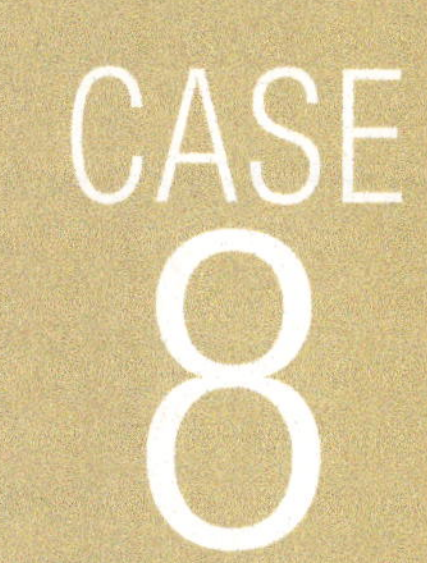

Chief Complaint

"Medication adjustment."

History of Present Illness

A 27-year-old male presents to the clinic seeking help in adjusting his psychiatric medications. He had been followed by your primary care partner; however, she is out of office on maternity leave. The patient reports he has had feelings of depression since high school but has never received a formal psychiatric diagnosis. Over the last year, he has found it difficult to function. One month ago, your partner prescribed him sertraline; the patient is uncertain if it has made any difference in his mood or energy level. He works as an EMT, with 12-hour shifts that vary in terms of daytime or overnight assignment. When returning home from work, he typically drinks a can of beer while absent mindedly scrolling through social media posts on his phone. After a shift, he feels like he does not even have the energy to change out of his uniform. Though he usually gets 6 to 8 hours of sleep at night, he has trouble falling asleep and does not feel ready to face the day upon waking, hitting the snooze button on his alarm at least a few times. The patient reports he recently shaved his head, explaining he does not always have time to shower in the morning before work. He takes naps on his days off, noting that he used to spend his free time going hiking or volunteering at a local animal rescue. He has started skipping meals, stating that he just does not feel hungry. On further query, he confesses that a person at the firehouse had commented on his weight, and since then, he has been embarrassed to change his clothes in the locker room. He then blurts out that he has developed feelings of attraction to this person, lamenting, "I don't know if that means I'm bisexual or what."

Review of Systems

The patient reports occasional headaches and back pain, which he attributes to the stress and physical exertion of his work. He also reports his libido has been reduced over the last few weeks. He has ordered some sildenafil from an online pharmacy but has not received it yet. He denies suicidal or homicidal ideation; however, he admits to a history of self-injury through cutting in high school and college. He denies having nightmares or nighttime awakenings.

Relevant History

He recalls attending a very bad car accident a few months ago—probably the most catastrophic he had seen in his young career as an EMT. He spoke with his supervisor afterward but did not feel the need to pursue counseling. He is uncertain if there is a family history of mental health issues, noting that this was not something typically discussed at home. Nonetheless, he suspects that his maternal grandmother took an antidepressant medication for a while after her husband died.

Allergies

His mother is allergic to penicillin and told him not to take it; no known food allergies.

Medications

- Melatonin 2mg PO QHS PRN
- Sertraline 25mg PO QAM.

Physical Examination

- *Vitals:* T 37°C (98.6°F), P 110, R 18, BP 142/89, SpO_2 100% on room air, Wt 136 kg (300 lb), Ht 193 cm (76 in.), BMI 36.5.
- *General:* Alert and active, not in acute distress. Appears stated age.
- *Eyes:* Normal conjunctiva without icterus. No exophthalmos. Wears eyeglasses.
- *Neck:* Supple. No cervical lymphadenopathy. No thyromegaly. Normal phonation.
- *Cardiovascular:* Tachycardic but otherwise normal rhythm with normal S1/S2 and no extra sounds.
- *Pulmonary:* CTA bilaterally without wheezes, rales, or rhonchi. Speaks in full sentences without breathlessness.
- *Gastrointestinal:* Obese, soft, nontender, with normoactive bowel sounds and no rebound or guarding. Faint, nonviolaceous striae. No apparent hepatomegaly, caput medusae, or ascites. No costovertebral angle tenderness or dullness on percussion.
- *Urogenital:* Exam deferred.
- *Skin:* Well-healed, linear scarring of the entire left anterior forearm and distal aspect of the medial left lower extremity, without keloid formation or apparent recent insult to skin integrity. No acanthosis nigricans noted in skin folds at the neck, axillae, or waist. Hair, skin, and nails are otherwise normal.
- *Psychiatric:* Pleasant and cooperative, A&O×3, quiet speech with depressed affect, inconsistent eye contact, slouched body posture, and fair insight. No hallucinations or delusions.
- *Neurologic:* No focal neurologic deficits, normal gait. Slowed speech.

Clinical Discussion Questions

1. What is the differential diagnosis?

2. What is the most likely diagnosis? Why?

3. Demonstrate your understanding about the pathophysiology of the most likely diagnosis.

4. Should tests/imaging studies be ordered? Which ones? Why? Think about tests/imaging beyond the primary care setting as well.

5. What are the next appropriate steps in management?

6. Review a reliable, recent source and demonstrate an understanding of the prevalence, prevention, and treatments. Provide references for your responses.

7. What are the pertinent ICD-10 and CPT (E/M) codes for this visit? Provide a short rationale.

8. What are the appropriate patient education topic for this case?

9. If not managed appropriately, what is/are the medical/legal concern(s) that may arise?

10. Think about interprofessional collaboration for this case. Provide a list of specialties or other disciplines and indicate what contribution these professionals might make to managing the patient.

BEDSIDE MANNER QUESTION

11. What would your communication style/approach be with this patient?

Answers available at courseconnect.springerpub.com.

CASE 9

THICK YELLOW TOENAILS, ADULT FEMALE

Chief Complaint

"Thick, yellow toenails."

History of Present Illness

A 64-year-old woman presents for her monthly check-in appointment. She has several chronic conditions that are well controlled through medications and she follows up with specialists involved in her care every 6 months. She is having surgery for a right rotator cuff tear later in the month and would like to discuss her thick, discolored toenails. She has had a number of health problems in the past 5 years requiring medication adjustments and surgeries, and now she believes she is "caught up" enough to get something done about her toenails. She reports her nails are very thick ("I haven't been able to cut my nails in years"), curled, and yellow. She saw a podiatrist about her hammertoe surgical repair last year, but she did not mention her toenails. She remembers having very "pretty" toenails in her 20s and 30s. She used to wear nail polish but stopped at least 20 years ago. She has never injured her toenails or wore high heels and does not remember ever having a fungal infection.

Review of Systems

The patient's ROS is positive for toenail discoloration and malformation. She denies rash or skin lesions on feet, limping, numbness, or tingling.

Relevant History

The patient's medical history is significant for T2DM, controlled with insulin and diet, and BL hammertoe of the great toes. Her surgical history includes a right carpal tunnel repair, BL bunionectomies, right shoulder rotator cuff repair, right trigger finger release, left shoulder arthroscopy, and right shoulder repair. She has a long history of chronic pain from rheumatoid arthritis and cervical and lumbar disc herniation, for which she is stable on chronic narcotics. The patient is married and on long-term disability because of multiple health problems. She is sexually active and lives with her husband and a roommate. Her exercise consists of a daily walk, using a walker, to the end of the driveway. Her family history is unknown as she was adopted as a toddler.

Allergies

No known drug or food allergies.

Medications

- Lantus 100 units/mL solution, Sig: 60 units QHS.
- Oxycodone hydrochloride 15 mg tablet, Sig: 1 tab PO Q6H PRN for pain.
- Sotalol 80 mg tablet, Sig: 1 tab PO BID.
- Rosuvastatin calcium 40 mg tablet, Sig: 1 tab PO QD.
- Citalopram 60 mg tablet, Sig: 1 tab PO QD.
- Amlodipine 5 mg tablet, Sig: 1 tab PO QD.
- Linagliptin 5 mg tablet, Sig: 1 tab PO QD.
- Aspirin enteric coated 81 mg delayed-release tablet, Sig: 1 tab PO QD.

Physical Examination

- *Vitals:* T 37°C (98.6°F), P 73, R 16, BP 118/72, HT 171.45 cm (67.5 in.), WT 120.6 kg (266 lb), BMI 41.04.
- *General:* Well-appearing woman, no acute distress, appears stated age, sitting comfortably in chair. Front-wheeled walker near chair.
- *Psychiatric:* Mildly anxious.
- *Skin, Hair, and Nails:* Skin normal in appearance; no rashes or lesions. Normal hair distribution, thin on top of scalp. Fingernails normal in color, texture, and shape; neatly trimmed to edge of nail bed, no cyanosis/clubbing. Toenails on BL feet deep yellow, thickened, and curved inward, extending beyond edge of toe.
- *Head:* Normal shape and appearance.
- *Lungs:* Clear in all lobes.
- *Heart:* RRR without murmur.
- *Neurologic:* A&O×3; color, sensation, and movement within normal limits on BL legs and feet.

Clinical Discussion Questions

1. What is the differential diagnosis?

2. What is the most likely diagnosis? Why?

3. Demonstrate your understanding about the pathophysiology of the most likely diagnosis.

4. Should tests/imaging studies be ordered? Which ones? Why? Think about tests/imaging beyond the primary care setting as well.

5. What are the next appropriate steps in management?

6. Review a credible research article(s) about this diagnosis. Demonstrate your understanding of the prevalence, diagnostic criteria, and treatment options. Include a list of your reference(s).

7. What are the pertinent ICD-10 and CPT (E/M) codes for this visit? Provide a short rationale.

8. What are the appropriate patient education topics for this case?

9. If not managed appropriately, what is/are the medical/legal concern(s) that may arise?

10. Think about interprofessional collaboration for this case. Provide a list of specialties or other disciplines and indicate what contribution these professionals might make to managing the patient.

BEDSIDE MANNER QUESTION

11. What would your communication style/approach be with this patient?

Answers available at courseconnect.springerpub.com.

MOOD CHANGES, ADULT MALE

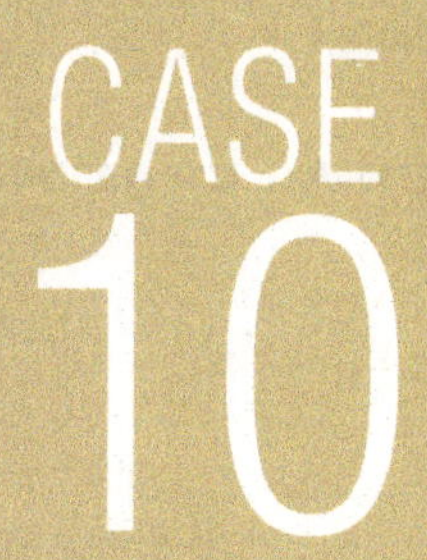

Chief Complaint

"Mood changes."

History of Present Illness

A 34-year-old man presents to a primary care office for evaluation of mood changes. He says he has been more easily agitated. The patient's husband has noted an increase in the patient's irritability and has asked him to be evaluated for depression. The patient has been treated for depression in the past. He denies current symptoms of depression but says he has been fatigued in the past year and has suffered frequent headaches. Despite exercising regularly, he has had weight gain, daytime fatigue, and joint pain.

His husband has also asked that he sleep in another room because of his snoring. The patient had been using a CPAP machine for OSA but finds the head strap increasingly uncomfortable to wear because of how tight it is despite attempts to adjust it. For this reason, he often does not use it. The patient recently had blood work done as part of a routine physical 3 weeks ago that found he was "prediabetic" and had elevated cholesterol.

The patient is also upset because he is no longer able to wear his wedding ring or a watch that was his father's, as they are now too small for him. He attributes this to the weight gain despite a healthy diet and regular exercise.

Review of Systems

The patient's ROS is positive for worsening peripheral vision, excessive sweating, fatigue, weight gain, headaches, sleep difficulties, change in mood, erectile dysfunction, skin darkening (around the neck and axilla), and joint pain.

The ROS is negative for bowel or bladder dysfunction, suicidal/homicidal ideation, head injury, change in appetite or thirst, seizures, loss of consciousness, numbness or tingling, involuntary movements or spasms, and abdominal pain.

Relevant History

The patient's medical history is significant for OSA, not controlled; hypertension; osteoarthritis of the right knee; and newly diagnosed prediabetes and hypercholesterolemia, which he is attempting to manage with lifestyle modifications. The patient denies alcohol, tobacco, or illicit drug use now or in the past. He has been married to the same man for 6 years, with no children and no siblings.

Allergies

No known drug allergies; no known food allergies.

Medications

- Hydrochlorothiazide 12.5 mg PO QD.
- Acetaminophen 1,000 mg PO QID PRN for knee pain.

PHYSICAL EXAMINATION

- *Vitals:* T 37.5°C (99.5°F), P 82, R 18, BP 142/86 mmHg, HT 190.5 cm (75 in.), WT 108.86 kg (240 lb), BMI 31.
- *General:* Well developed, well nourished, no acute distress.
- *Psychiatric:* Able to maintain attention and answer questions; PHQ-9 score 6 (mild depression, affirmative answers only to "feeling tired" and "trouble staying asleep").
- *Skin, Hair, and Nails:* Dense facial hair distribution, velvety darkening of the skin around the neck and axilla; skin is moist diffusely, most specifically in the hands.
- *Head:* Thickset jaw, protruding brow line.
- *Eyes:* Mildly diminished peripheral vision on visual fields by confrontation bilaterally; EOMs intact in six cardinal positions of gaze; PERRLA bilaterally.
- *ENT/Mouth:* Slight gap between two front teeth; hypertrophy of pharyngeal soft tissues.
- *Neck:* No abnormalities of thyroid on palpation.
- *Lungs:* CTA bilaterally.
- *Heart:* No murmurs, gallops, or rubs; RRR; PMI displaced laterally.
- *Genital/Rectal:* Deferred.
- *Musculoskeletal:* Prominence of bony structures in joints of hands, upper extremities, and lower extremities; widened joints and enlarged soft tissue structure around multiple joints; slight hypermobility in joints of upper and lower extremities as noted on ROS evaluation; crepitus present in BL knees on flexion and extension; hands and feet are enlarged (widened) compared proportionately to the height of the patient.
- *Neurologic:* Sensation intact to light and sharp touch in the upper and lower extremities; strength 5/5 in the upper and lower extremities bilaterally; DTRs 2+ for tricep, bicep, brachioradialis, patellar, and Achilles reflexes bilaterally; negative Babinski sign; no increased or decreased tone on passive movement of the limbs.

CLINICAL DISCUSSION QUESTIONS

1. What is the differential diagnosis?

____

____

____

____

2. What is the most likely diagnosis? Why?

____

____

____

____

3. Demonstrate your understanding about the pathophysiology of the most likely diagnosis.

____

____

____

____

4. Should tests/imaging studies be ordered? Which ones? Why? Think about tests/imaging beyond the primary care setting as well.

5. What are the next appropriate steps in management?

6. Review a recent and credible research article(s) about this diagnosis. Demonstrate your understanding of the underlying causes, associated conditions, and complications. Include a list of your reference(s).

7. What are the pertinent ICD-10 and CPT (E/M) codes for this visit? Provide a short rationale.

8. What are the appropriate patient education topics for this case?

9. If not managed appropriately, what is/are the medical/legal concern(s) that may arise?

10. Think about interprofessional collaboration for this case. Provide a list of specialties or other disciplines and indicate what contribution these professionals might make to managing the patient.

BEDSIDE MANNER QUESTIONS

11. What would your communication style/approach be with this patient?

12. If a patient is distressed by the diagnosis, what might offer support?

Answers available at courseconnect.springerpub.com.

CASE 11

VAGINAL BLEEDING AND SPOTTING, ADULT FEMALE

Chief Complaint

"Vaginal bleeding/spotting."

History of Present Illness

A 41-year-old female presents with over 1 year of vaginal bleeding and spotting in between her periods as well as after sexual intercourse. Initially, her symptoms were occasional; however, for the last 3 to 4 months, she reports consistent spotting in between her menstrual periods, heavier periods, and significant bleeding consistently after sexual intercourse. The patient has been sexually active with one male partner for the last 5 years and she denies any new partners. The patient reports a history of chlamydia infection a few years ago but it was reportedly treated. She reports negative STI testing within the past year. Prior to the last year, she denies any history of dyspareunia, heavy periods, or intermenstrual spotting. The patient also denies any current or prior physical or sexual abuse/trauma.

Review of Systems

The patient's ROS is currently negative for uterine cramping, abdominal pain, nausea, vomiting, fevers, or chills. The patient denies current breast tenderness and dizziness or lightheadedness.

Relevant History

The patient experienced menarche at age 12 with initially irregular periods for a few years. By the age of 17, she had regular, monthly periods up until the last year. The patient has never been pregnant and denies any abortions or miscarriages. She is currently using condoms consistently as contraception.

She reports she has just moved to the area from New York and her last Pap smear was 3 years ago, reportedly normal. She denies any history of abnormal Pap smears.

The patient's medical history is significant for T2DM, well-controlled with diet. Last Hgb A1C was 6.7%, less than 3 months ago.

Allergies

No known drug allergies; no known food allergies

Medications

None.

Physical Examination

- *Vitals:* T 35.8°C (96.5°F), P 81, R 18, BP 127/86, HT 160 cm (63 in.), WT 81.6 kg (180 lb), BMI 31.9.
- *General:* Appears to be in no acute distress.
- *Lungs:* CTA bilaterally without rales, rhonchi, wheezing, or diminished breath sounds.
- *Heart:* RRR. Normal S1 and S2. No S3, S4, or murmurs. No carotid bruits. No peripheral edema, cyanosis, or pallor.

- *Abdomen:* Soft, nondistended, nontender. No guarding or rebound. No masses palpated. Positive BS.
- *Genital/Rectal:* Normally developed external female genitalia with no external lesions or eruptions. Vagina without any lesions, lacerations, or trauma noted. Cervix noted to have an exophytic friable, "cauliflower-like" mass between 4 o'clock and 6 o'clock, unable to visualize uterine os.

Clinical Discussion Questions

1. What is the differential diagnosis?

2. What is the most likely diagnosis? Why?

3. Demonstrate your understanding about the pathophysiology of the most likely diagnosis.

4. Should tests/imaging studies be ordered? Which ones? Why? Think about tests/imaging beyond the primary care setting as well.

5. What are the next appropriate steps in management?

6. What are the risk factors, causes, and most common site for this diagnosis? Provide references for your response.

7. What are the pertinent ICD-10 and CPT (E/M) codes for this visit? Provide a short rationale.

8. What are the appropriate patient education topics for this case?

9. If not managed appropriately, what is/are the medical/legal concern(s) that may arise?

10. Think about interprofessional collaboration for this case. Provide a list of specialties or other disciplines and indicate what contribution these professionals might make to managing the patient.

BEDSIDE MANNER QUESTIONS

11. How would you communicate your likely diagnosis to the patient?

12. If the patient shows distress at what you communicate, how would you provide support?

____

____

____

____

Answers available at courseconnect.springerpub.com.

CASE 12

BURNING WITH URINATION, ADULT MALE

Chief Complaint

"Burning with urination."

History of Present Illness

A 21-year-old man presents as a new patient for an evaluation of burning with urination for 3 days. He states he noticed it to be mild at first and thought maybe it was just irritation from a new soap he was using, but then it worsened. He also notes a small amount of clear penile discharge. When he had these same symptoms a few months ago, he went to a local DOH and was given antibiotics but does not remember the drug's name. His symptoms went away immediately after treatment then, and he has been fine until this present concern. The patient's sexual history reveals he is active with both women and men but predominantly men. He has no current primary sexual partner, and he states having about five male sexual partners in the past 3 months. When he does have sex with men, he states he is primarily a "top" (insertive) partner with anal sex and both gives and receives oral sex. He says he sometimes does and sometimes does not use condoms with anal sex, depending on how much he trusts his sexual partner, and never uses condoms with oral sex. His last HIV test was 4 months ago during a student testing initiative; it was negative.

Review of Systems

Positive ROS findings as noted in the HPI. The ROS is negative for fever, chills, SOB, chest pain, abdominal pain, or rash.

Relevant History

The patient's medical history is significant for mild intermittent reactive airway disease controlled with an albuterol inhaler PRN. He uses an inhaler only occasionally, about once every couple of months. He is a social drinker at parties on weekends, rarely smokes or ingests marijuana, and has no history of tobacco use or vaping. He has had no surgeries and is a senior in college with plans to pursue a PhD when he graduates. He denies any experimentation or use of other substances like methamphetamines, cocaine, opiates, or others. His family history is noncontributory.

Allergies

No known drug allergies; no known food allergies.

Medications

Albuterol inhaler 2 puffs every 4 to 6 hours PRN.

Physical Examination

- *Vitals:* T 36°C (97°F), P 82, R 12, BP 113/82, WT 100.7 kg (222 lb), HT 180.3 cm (71 in.), BMI 31.
- *General:* Thin male in no acute distress.
- *Psychiatric:* Slightly anxious behavior noted.
- *Skin, Hair, and Nails:* No notable rashes or lesions.

- *Abdomen:* Soft, nontender, not distended, active BS, no masses felt.
- *Genital/Rectal:* Uncircumcised male, able to retract foreskin easily. Clear discharge when instructed to milk the shaft. No lesions or rashes noted. Shotty inguinal lymphadenopathy noted, scrotum with mild tenderness when palpating left testicle. Both testicles are smooth with no evidence of masses or nodules. Valsalva maneuver reveals no hernia on either side. Rectal exam deferred.

CLINICAL DISCUSSION QUESTIONS

1. What is the differential diagnosis?

2. What is the most likely diagnosis? Why?

3. Demonstrate your understanding about the pathophysiology of the most likely diagnosis.

4. Should tests/imaging studies be ordered? Which ones? Why? Think about tests/imaging beyond the primary care setting as well.

5. What are the next appropriate steps in management?

6. What are the testing recommendations, treatment options, and screening guidelines for this diagnosis? Provide references for your response.

7. What are the pertinent ICD-10 and CPT (E/M) codes for this visit? Provide a short rationale.

8. What are the appropriate patient education topics for this case?

9. If not managed appropriately, what is/are the medical/legal concern(s) that may arise?

10. Think about interprofessional collaboration for this case. Provide a list of specialties or other disciplines and indicate what contribution these professionals might make to managing the patient.

BEDSIDE MANNER QUESTIONS

11. What would your communication style/approach be with this patient?

12. If a patient is distressed by the diagnosis, what might offer support?

Answers available at courseconnect.springerpub.com.

CASE 13

CONSTIPATION, ADULT FEMALE

Chief Complaint

"Constipation."

History of Present Illness

A 58-year-old woman with a complicated history of chronic low back pain, bipolar disorder, mixed anxiety, and depressive disorder presents to her PCP, a PA, complaining of constipation for several months. Constipation has been intermittent and has gotten worse over the past few weeks. She is now having a bowel movement about once every 4 days; her stools are hard and painful, and she has bright red blood on the toilet paper after she wipes. She does not feel she is able to completely evacuate her bowels. She denies melena, abdominal pain, bloating or excessive gas, loose stools, or fecal incontinence. She is afraid to take medications and has not tried any OTC treatments for fear of side effects. She has had no changes in her regular medications and no short-acting narcotics for breakthrough pain. She reports a regular diet (lean protein, fruits/vegetables, and grains) without changes; she admits to not drinking enough water, about 20 ounces daily; and she denies caffeine or alcohol use. Her stress level has not increased; she admits to daily anxiety that limits her activities and reports anxiety is at baseline. She has never had a colonoscopy due to anxiety about the procedure and potential outcomes. Her chronic low back pain has been stable for the past 6 years with current medications; she has been on the same dose of extended-release morphine sulfate for 4 years. She fears discontinuing morphine sulfate will result in worsened back pain. She does not exercise, does not receive physical therapy, and is not followed by pain management.

Review of Systems

The patient's ROS is positive for constipation, bright red blood per rectum, and anxiety. The ROS is negative for fever, night sweats, weight changes, and fatigue; hair or skin changes; heat or cold intolerance; and belching, halitosis, heartburn, early satiety, nausea, or vomiting. The patient was also negative for chest pain, palpitations, SOB, mania, ideas of grandiosity, hallucinations, suicidal ideations, and worsening anxiety or panic.

Relevant History

The patient's medical history is significant for asthma (since childhood), bipolar disorder (age 25), mixed anxiety and depressive disorder (age 45), GERD (age 50), hyperlipidemia (age 52), hypothyroidism secondary to lithium use (age 42; TSH last checked 3 months ago, in normal range), IBS-C (age 48), chronic low back pain (age 52), psoriasis (age 23), diverticulitis (last episode 2 years ago, diet controlled), and primary hyperparathyroidism with hypercalcemia post partial resection 15 months ago (serum calcium level in normal range 3 months ago). Her social history includes no use of alcohol, tobacco, or recreational drugs. She is married with no children; she volunteers at her church, sings in the choir, and performs charity work with older people. Her family history is noncontributory.

Allergies

Penicillin (hives); no known food allergies.

Medications

- Levothyroxine 75 mcg PO QD.
- Omeprazole, extended release, 40 mg PO QD.

- Morphine sulfate, extended release, 60 mg PO QD.
- Lithium 300 mg, PO QD.
- Clonazepam 1 mg PO QHS PRN for insomnia/anxiety.
- Desonide 0.05% topical ointment, apply sparingly to affected area(s) BID.
- Albuterol inhaler, inhale two puffs Q4h PRN for wheezing and dyspnea.

PHYSICAL EXAMINATION

- *Vitals:* T 37°C (98.6°F), P 76, R 12, BP 115/74, HT 152 cm (60 in.), WT 62 kg (138 lb), BMI 27.
- *General:* Well-developed, well-nourished female in no apparent distress.
- *Psychiatric:* Anxious, no pressured speech, good eye contact, good insight, no suicidal ideation.
- *Skin, Hair, and Nails:* Mild psoriasis in ears, scalp; skin is warm and dry, no edema or rash; no hair or eyebrow thinning; no nail pits or splitting.
- *Neck:* Well-healed scar from parathyroid surgery, normal thyroid/neck exam.
- *Lungs:* CTA bilaterally.
- *Heart:* RRR, no murmurs, rubs, or gallops; no peripheral edema.
- *Abdomen:* Soft, nontender, nondistended, active BS in all quadrants, no hepatosplenomegaly or masses.
- *Musculoskeletal:* Lumbosacral region without tenderness or muscle spasm, LROM in lumbar spine.
- *Neurologic:* Lower extremity sensation intact, DTR 2+ patella, Achilles; negative SLR bilaterally.

CLINICAL DISCUSSION QUESTIONS

1. What is the differential diagnosis?

2. What is the most likely diagnosis? Why?

3. Demonstrate your understanding about the pathophysiology of the most likely diagnosis.

4. Should tests/imaging studies be ordered? Which ones? Why? Think about tests/imaging beyond the primary care setting as well.

5. What are the next appropriate steps in management?

6. What are the treatment options for this diagnosis? Provide references for your response.

7. What are the pertinent ICD-10 and CPT (E/M) codes for this visit? Provide a short rationale.

8. What is the appropriate patient education topic for this case?

9. If not managed appropriately, what is/are the medical/legal concern(s) that may arise?

10. Think about interprofessional collaboration for this case. Provide a list of specialties or other disciplines and indicate what contribution these professionals might make to managing the patient.

Bedside Manner Questions

11. What would your communication style/approach be with this patient?

12. If a patient is distressed by the diagnosis, what might offer support?

Answers available at courseconnect.springerpub.com.

FATIGUE AND GENERAL MALAISE, ADULT MALE

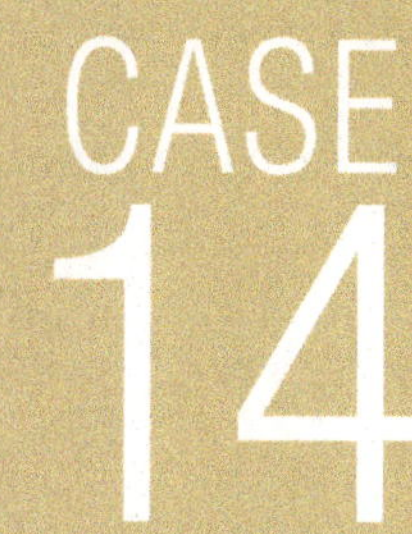

Chief Complaint

"Fatigue, general malaise."

History of Present Illness

A 55-year-old man presents to his PCP with his wife after a 4-hour history of "feeling bad." This began suddenly while at home. He feels tired and does not want to do anything other than sit in his chair. He is winded quickly when he is moving around and feels like he has an upset stomach and believes it is indigestion. However, his wife notes he is not himself and she is worried about him. Upon further questioning, he does state he has pain and it is more over his chest than his abdomen. It does not radiate to his arm or neck. He has a hard time rating the pain, stating, "It just hurts." His best description of the pain is that it is dull. Sitting in his recliner seems to ease his pain. He is on hydrocodone/acetaminophen 10/325 mg for chronic lower back pain, and this has not relieved his current symptoms. He has not wanted to eat anything today due to fatigue. His wife also notes he appears sweaty even though he has not done much all day.

The patient admits he has not been faithfully checking his BP as he was asked to do on a prior visit. When he does check, which is approximately once a week, it is in the range of 140 to 150 for systolic; he does not know his diastolic BP. His last cholesterol level was checked 4 months ago, and his LDL was mildly elevated at 140; total cholesterol, HDL, and triglycerides were within normal limits.

Review of Systems

The patient's ROS is positive for fatigue, loss of appetite, chest pain, SOB on exertion, anxiety, and chronic lower back pain. The review is negative for fever, rhinorrhea, sore throat, ear pain, palpitations, edema of the lower legs, orthopnea, wheezing, stridor, cough, nausea and vomiting, diarrhea, constipation, neck pain/stiffness, gait problems, depression, hallucinations, loss of consciousness, numbness, or weakness.

Relevant History

The patient's medical history includes hypercholesterolemia, HTN, obesity, chronic lower-back pain, and generalized anxiety. He had a lumbar discectomy at age 44. He lives with his wife; they are happily married. He is sexually active and in a monogamous relationship with his wife. He drinks a few beers over the weekend and says he quit smoking 10 years ago but has a 1-pack-per-day history for 20 years. He admits to marijuana usage about a month ago. His father was diagnosed with CAD at an unknown age and is deceased.

Allergies

No known drug allergies; no known food allergies.

Medications

- Atorvastatin 10 mg PO QD.
- Hydrocodone/acetaminophen 10/325 mg PO QID PRN.
- Lisinopril 10 mg PO QD.
- Alprazolam 0.5 mg PO QID PRN.

PHYSICAL EXAMINATION

- *Vitals:* T 37°C (98.6°F), P 94, R 16, BP 140/85, SpO_2 95%, WT 117 kg (258 lb), HT 177.8 cm (70 in.), BMI 37.
- *General:* Appears sweaty and uncomfortable. Patient is obese.
- *Psychiatric:* Anxious.
- *Skin, Hair, and Nails:* Cool to touch and damp, pink, no pallor noted. No abnormal findings with hair or nails.
- *Lungs:* Breathing is nonlabored. He is not using accessory muscles for breathing, and there are no retractions noted. Lung fields are CTA bilaterally with good air movement; no wheezes, crackles, or rales noted.
- *Heart:* RRR, no murmur or extra sounds noted. Chest is nontender to palpation.
- *Vascular:* Radial and pedal pulses are 2+ bilaterally. He has a capillary refill time of <2 seconds in his fingers and toes. There is no edema noted in his extremities. No cyanosis is noted around the mouth or in extremities. JVD is not noted.
- *Abdomen:* BS normal. Soft, nontender, no distension.
- *Neurologic:* Cranial nerves II to XII grossly intact. Patient is A&O×3.

CLINICAL DISCUSSION QUESTIONS

1. What is the differential diagnosis?

2. What is the most likely diagnosis? Why?

3. Demonstrate your understanding about the pathophysiology of the most likely diagnosis.

4. Should tests/imaging studies be ordered? Which ones? Why? Think about tests/imaging beyond the primary care setting as well.

5. What are the next appropriate steps in management?

6. What are the risk predictors and symptom duration of the diagnosis? Provide references for your response.

7. What are the pertinent ICD-10 and CPT (E/M) codes for this visit? Provide a short rationale.

8. What is the appropriate patient education topic for this case?

9. If not managed appropriately, what is/are the medical/legal concern(s) that may arise?

10. Think about interprofessional collaboration for this case. Provide a list of specialties or other disciplines and indicate what contribution these professionals might make to managing the patient.

BEDSIDE MANNER QUESTIONS

11. What would your communication style/approach be with this patient and his wife?

12. If a patient and his wife are distressed by a diagnosis, what might offer support?

Answers available at courseconnect.springerpub.com.

CASE 15

DIZZINESS AND DIFFICULTY HEARING, ADULT MALE

Chief Complaint

"Dizziness and hearing difficulty."

History of Present Illness

A 64-year-old man presents to his PCP complaining of intermittent episodes of dizziness occurring over the past year. The dizziness, described as a spinning sensation, comes every 1 to 2 weeks and generally lasts for 6 to 12 hours. These episodes are often accompanied by nausea and vomiting. He has more recently noticed hearing fluctuations, especially in his left ear. The hearing loss is worse just before and during attacks and then improves. He also now describes a sense of aural fullness and tinnitus, described as a low-frequency blowing or roaring sound in the ear, associated with the episodes. He attributes these symptoms to noise exposure with his work. He has taken OTC meclizine to help with the dizziness, with some relief of the symptoms.

Review of Systems

The patient's ROS is positive for vertigo, tinnitus, hearing loss, nausea, and vomiting. He has occasional headaches that respond to treatment with acetaminophen. His ROS is negative for fever, chills, weight loss, or fatigue.

Relevant History

The patient has had no major illnesses, injuries, surgeries, or hospitalizations. He is a lifelong nonsmoker and drinks one to two glasses of wine per week. He is employed as a high school music teacher and plays in a band part-time on weekends. The patient is married and has three grown children who are all in good health. His family history is significant for HTN in both parents. There is no family history of cancer, early heart disease, or DM.

Allergies

No known medical allergies; no known drug allergies.

Medications

- Meclizine 25 mg PO TID OTC, PRN.
- Acetaminophen, 500 mg PRN.

Physical Examination

- *Vitals:* T 37°C (98.6°F), P 76, R 14, BP 132/82, HT 177.8 cm (70 in.), WT 81.65 kg (180 lb), BMI 25.8.
- *General:* Well-developed and nourished 64-year-old male patient in no acute distress.
- *Psychiatric:* Appears mildly anxious.
- *Skin, Hair, and Nails:* Skin warm and dry, no rashes or bleeding tendency. No abnormal findings with hair or nails.
- *ENT/Mouth:* TMs appear pearly, gray with no fluid noted. Hearing is decreased in the left ear as compared to the right on gross testing. Oral mucosa is moist; dentition in good repair with no caries or erosions.

- *Neck:* Supple with no adenopathy or thyroid enlargement.
- *Lungs:* CTA bilaterally.
- *Heart:* RRR, without murmur, gallop, or rub.
- *Abdomen:* Soft with no masses, organomegaly, or tenderness. Active BS heard in all quadrants.
- *Neurologic:* A&O×3; immediate, recent, and remote memory intact; Cranial nerves II–XII grossly intact; strength 3/5 and DTRs 2+ symmetrical in all extremities; sensation, coordination, balance, cerebellar function, and gait intact.

Clinical Discussion Questions

1. What is the differential diagnosis?

2. What is the most likely diagnosis? Why?

3. Demonstrate your understanding about the pathophysiology of the most likely diagnosis.

4. Should tests/imaging studies be ordered? Which ones? Why? Think about tests/imaging beyond the primary care setting as well.

5. What are the next appropriate steps in management?

6. What are the diagnostic criteria and treatment options for this diagnosis? Provide references for your response.

7. What are the pertinent ICD-10 and CPT (E/M) codes for this visit? Provide a short rationale.

8. What is the appropriate patient education for this case?

9. If not managed appropriately, what is/are the medical/legal concern(s) that may arise?

10. Think about interprofessional collaboration for this case. Provide a list of specialties or other disciplines and indicate what contribution these professionals might make to managing the patient.

BEDSIDE MANNER QUESTION

11. What would be your communication style/approach with this patient?

Answers available at courseconnect.springerpub.com.

CASE 16

BAD HEADACHE, ADULT FEMALE

Chief Complaint

"Bad headache."

History of Present Illness

A 48-year-old woman presents to her PCP with a 2-day history of a bad headache. She asks the lights to be turned off in the exam room to lessen the pain. Her pain began yesterday morning, an hour after awakening. She reports seeing "zigzags of lights" in her vision for several minutes before the headache began and grew over 2 hours. She rated the pain as 8/10 initially and now rates it as 5/10. She points to her left temple and states it is an "intense, steady pain." She reports nausea with two episodes of vomiting yesterday, with a more throbbing pain that made it difficult to sleep. Taking 1,000 mg acetaminophen helps, but any relief only lasts a couple of hours. She has had this type of headache before (including the visual disturbance) but it never lasted this long. Her last headache was about a month ago, lasting less than a day. The patient is a graduate student in her third of five semesters, lives with an older sister, and works as a barista in the evenings and on weekends. She cannot work or study with this headache. She is on oral birth control but on no other medications and admits to increased stress due to finances, a fight with her boyfriend, and intense studies.

Review of Systems

The patient's ROS is positive for headache, nausea/vomiting, and visual changes. Significant negatives are an absence of fever, congestion, dizziness, or extremity weakness.

Relevant History

The patient is "generally healthy" and denies recent illness. By clinic record, her only surgery was a laparoscopic appendectomy at age 13 with no complications. She reports two to three beers/week and smokes marijuana one to two times a month. Her parents are divorced; her mother has T2DM and her father has HTN and prostate cancer (under treatment). Her mother has always had similar headaches, saying, "There's nothing that can be done but to wait it out." There is no family history of cranial bleeding or other cancers.

Allergies

No known medical allergies; no known food allergies.

Medications

1,000 mg acetaminophen PRN.

Physical Examination

- *Vitals:* T 37°C (98.6°F), P 84, R 18, BP 110/70, HT 157.5 cm (62 in.), WT 60.8 kg (134 lb), BMI 24.5.
- *General:* Moderate distress consistent with chief complaint, well-nourished, cooperative adult.
- *Psychiatric:* Appropriate concern for health.
- *Skin, Hair, and Nails:* No rashes or lesions. No abnormal findings with hair or nails.
- *Eyes:* PERRLA, visual fields full, fundi negative for hemorrhages, disc margins sharp.

- *Lungs:* CTA bilaterally.
- *Heart:* RRR without murmur.
- *Abdomen:* Soft without tenderness, no hepatomegaly, spleen/kidneys not palpable.
- *Neurologic:* A&O×3, CN II–XII grossly intact, Romberg negative, extremity DTRs 2+/4+, muscle strength symmetrically equal in extremities.

CLINICAL DISCUSSION QUESTIONS

1. What is the differential diagnosis?

2. What is the most likely diagnosis? Why?

3. Demonstrate your understanding about the pathophysiology of the most likely diagnosis.

4. Should tests/imaging studies be ordered? Which ones? Why? Think about tests/imaging beyond the primary care setting as well.

5. What are the next appropriate steps in management?

6. What are the diagnostic criteria and treatment options for this diagnosis? Provide references for your response.

7. What are the pertinent ICD-10 and CPT (E/M) codes for this visit? Provide a short rationale.

8. What is the appropriate patient education topic for this case?

9. If not managed appropriately, what is/are the medical/legal concern(s) that may arise?

10. Think about interprofessional collaboration for this case. Provide a list of specialties or other disciplines and indicate what contribution these professionals might make to managing the patient.

BEDSIDE MANNER QUESTION

11. What would be your communication style/approach with this patient?

Answers available at courseconnect.springerpub.com.

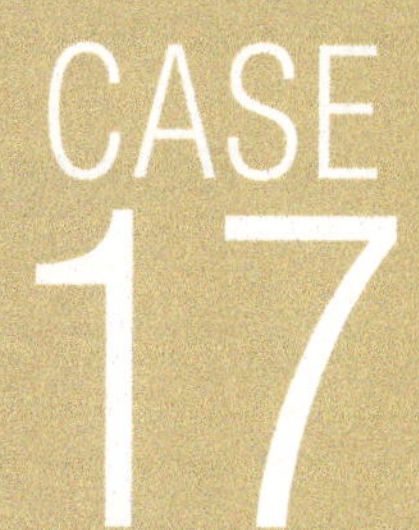

ABDOMINAL PAIN, ADULT FEMALE

Chief Complaint

"Abdominal pain."

History of present Illness

A 53-year-old woman presents with complaints of gnawing and constant 6/10 abdominal pain that started the day prior. She states she is afraid to eat anything for fear the pain will worsen. She reports an episode similar to this occurring 5 years ago after returning home from overseas travel. She recalls being told by a physician that she probably had food poisoning, being given an antibiotic, and feeling better 2 to 3 days later. She says this has not happened since. She cannot think of anything she may have eaten that could have caused this pain, as it "came out of nowhere." Her last meal was a breakfast of rye toast and yogurt with blackberries yesterday.

She reports being very feverish, sweaty, and nauseated when the pain first started. She denies vomiting but does admit to a few of bouts of dry heaves. She is unable to point to where it hurts the most, stating, "It's all over." She admits to feeling bloated and having multiple bowel movements, with her last one just prior to presentation. She states her stools have gone from soft to loose, thin ribbons, and now to nothing at all. She feels a need to evacuate her bowels, but nothing comes out. She worries about having bloody stools similar to those she had 5 years ago but has not seen that yet. She denies dysuria. She admits to having a high-stress job but denies ever being diagnosed with IBS or IBD. She has not traveled recently, nor has she been around anyone with similar symptoms. Her last colonoscopy was 5 years ago and was unremarkable.

Review of Systems

The patient's ROS is positive for subjective fever with chills, diaphoresis, difficulty sleeping due to abdominal pain, dry mouth, GERD, and reduced appetite. She denies recent unintentional weight loss or gain. Her ROS is negative for trouble swallowing, rectal bleeding, black or tarry stools, excessive belching or passing gas, liver problems, hepatitis, and jaundice.

Relevant History

The patient has a history of GERD, biliary dyskinesia with resultant laparoscopic cholecystectomy, uterine fibroids with resultant total abdominal hysterectomy, nephrolithiasis, and menopause. She drinks one to two glasses of wine with dinner 2 to 3 nights a week. Her family history is noncontributory.

Allergies

Erythromycin (hives); no known food allergies.

Medications

- Pantoprazole 40 mg PO QD.
- Calcium 600 mg PO BID.
- Vitamin D 800 IU PO BID.

PHYSICAL EXAMINATION

- *Vitals:* T 37.7°C (99.8°F), P 86, R 14, BP 146/94, HT 173 cm (68 in.), WT 76 kg (168 lb), BMI 25.5.
- *General:* Well-dressed and well-nourished female who appears younger than stated age, in obvious discomfort laying in the fetal position on the examination table. She is A&O.
- *Eyes:* Nonicteric, sclera injected, conjunctiva pink bilaterally. PERRLA.
- *ENT/Mouth:* Dry mucosa, no lesions, patent oropharynx, 1+ BL tonsils pink without exudate, uvula midline.
- *Neck:* Supple, anterior cervical lymphadenopathy bilaterally.
- *Lungs:* CTA bilaterally.
- *Heart:* +S1/S2, RRR, without murmurs, rubs, or gallops.
- *Peripheral Vascular:* Warm throughout, all pulses 2+ symmetric bilaterally, capillary refill time <2 seconds throughout.
- *Abdomen:* Distended abdomen; well-healed surgical scars in the mid-epigastric region, RUQ, and suprapubic region. Hyperactive BS ×4; diffusely tender mid to LLQ with rebound tenderness; no thrills, no bruits, no costovertebral angle tenderness.
- *Genital/Rectal:* (+) rectal tone, (+) guaiac, no external hemorrhoids.
- *Neurologic:* Cranial nerves II to XII grossly intact, speech and gait appropriate.

CLINICAL DISCUSSION QUESTIONS

1. What is the differential diagnosis?

2. What is the most likely diagnosis? Why?

3. Demonstrate your understanding about the pathophysiology of the most likely diagnosis.

4. Should tests/imaging studies be ordered? Which ones? Why? Think about tests/imaging beyond the primary care setting as well.

5. What are the next appropriate steps in management?

6. Review a reliable, recent reference regarding risk factors and treatment approaches for this diagnosis. Provide references for your response.

7. What are the pertinent ICD-10 and CPT (E/M) codes for this visit? Provide a short rationale.

8. What are appropriate patient education topics for this case?

9. If not managed appropriately, what is/are the medical/legal concern(s) that may arise?

10. Think about interprofessional collaboration for this case. Provide a list of specialties or other disciplines and indicate what contribution these professionals might make to managing the patient.

BEDSIDE MANNER QUESTION

11. What would your communication style/approach be with this patient?

Answers available at courseconnect.springerpub.com.

CASE 18

PAINFUL URINATION, ADULT MALE

Chief Complaint

"Painful urination."

History of Present Illness

A 32-year-old single man presents to his PCP with complaints of dysuria for the past week. He reports 8/10 burning with a painfully heavy sensation in his bladder and rectum, and he is unable to void except small amounts with great frequency throughout the day. He also complains of nocturia, which he denies ever occurred before. He reports a fever of 38.2°C (100.7°F) with chills that started yesterday. He admits to discomfort with bowel movements and is trying hard not to strain as the pain intensifies. He discloses having multiple female sexual partners and seldom uses condoms but relies on his partners to provide birth control. He was last sexually active 4 to 5 days ago, engaging in unprotected anal intercourse. He denies ever having STIs; blood in his urine, ejaculate, or stool; penile discharge or pain; abdominal pain; and scrotal or testicular pain. He has not tried any OTC medications to relieve his pain or fever.

Review of Systems

The patient's ROS is positive for increased frequency of urination with burning pain/pressure, nocturia, urgency, reduced caliber of stream, and hesitancy. He admits to fever, chills, malaise, and insomnia. His ROS is negative for nausea, vomiting, abdominal pain, changes in bowel movement, rectal bleeding, hemorrhoids, constipation, diarrhea, or hepatitis. He denies kidney stones, hernias, penile discharge, lesions, testicular pain, masses, STIs, or exposure to HIV.

Relevant History

The patient has a history of hypercholesterolemia. He has smoked a pack of cigarettes a day for 10 years. He consumes 3 to 4 alcoholic drinks on the weekends. He denies any recreational or illicit drug use.

Allergies

No known drug allergies; no known food allergies.

Medications

Atorvastatin 20 mg PO QD.

Physical Examination

- *Vitals:* T 38.4°C (101.2°F), P 104, R 14, BP 148/92, HT 188 cm (74 in.), WT 100.2 kg (221 lb), BMI 28.4.
- *General:* Well-developed, well-nourished male appearing of stated age laying in obvious discomfort on the examination table. He is alert and oriented, makes good eye contact, and answers all questions appropriately.
- *Skin, Hair, and Nails:* Consistently warm throughout; diaphoretic; without rashes, lesions, or masses.
- *ENT/Mouth:* Good repair of teeth and gums, no bleeding. Dry mucosa without lesions or masses, patent oropharynx, uvula midline.
- *Neck:* FROM, supple, anterior cervical and tonsillar adenopathy bilaterally.

- *Lungs:* CTA bilaterally, without wheezes.
- *Heart:* +S1/S2, RRR, without murmurs, rubs, or gallops.
- *Abdomen:* Protuberant, soft, BS×4, tender at suprapubic aspect. Negative CVA tenderness.
- *Genital/Rectal:* Circumcised male without urethral discharge, no scrotal masses, lesions or varicosities. (++) perineal pain, prostate firm, unable to determine the size (performed gently), hot to the touch, no masses, guaiac (−).
- *Musculoskeletal:* FROM throughout without pain.
- *Neurologic:* Cranial nerves II to XII grossly intact.

CLINICAL DISCUSSION QUESTIONS

1. What is the differential diagnosis?

2. What is the most likely diagnosis? Why?

3. Demonstrate your understanding about the pathophysiology of the most likely diagnosis.

4. Should tests/imaging studies be ordered? Which ones? Why? Think about tests/imaging beyond the primary care setting as well.

5. What are the next appropriate steps in management?

6. What are the prevalence, risk factors, typical presentation, and complications of this diagnosis? Provide references for your response.

7. What are the pertinent ICD-10 and CPT (E/M) codes for this visit? Provide a short rationale.

8. What is the appropriate patient education topic for this case?

9. If not managed appropriately, what is/are the medical/legal concern(s) that may arise?

10. Think about interprofessional collaboration for this case. Provide a list of specialties or other disciplines and indicate what contribution these professionals might make to managing the patient.

BEDSIDE MANNER QUESTION

11. What would your communication style/approach be with this patient?

Answers available at courseconnect.springerpub.com.

CASE 19

BLURRED VISION IN THE LEFT EYE, ADULT FEMALE

Chief Complaint

"Blurred vision in the left eye."

History of Present Illness

A 63-year-old White woman with a history of HTN, DM, and myopia presents to her PCP with an acute onset of blurred vision in the OS. She stated that it seemed like "a curtain came down over my eye" and was progressively getting worse by the time she arrived at the clinic. She was wearing dark glasses to relieve the discomfort from sunlight. Prior to her blurred vision, she experienced flashes of light and floaters in the eye. The patient was anxious and worried about permanent vision loss.

Review of Systems

The patient's ROS is positive for blurred vision, flashes, floaters, and mild photophobia in the OS. Her ROS is negative for pain, double vision, halos, or eye redness. She denies fever, chills, headaches, diarrhea, vomiting, or weight change. The patient denies other HEENT symptoms such as hearing defects and nostril or sinus problems. Her cardiopulmonary systems were unremarkable. She has no chest pain, SOB, palpitations, or extremity edema. A neurologic ROS is negative for dizziness, confusion, gait imbalances, or extremity weakness.

Relevant History

The patient has a history of HTN (diagnosed at age 50 and well controlled by lifestyle and antihypertensives). She has a history of poorly controlled T2DM (diagnosed at age 55) and was taking oral antidiabetic drugs (last Hgb A1C was 7.8). Other medical conditions included myopia diagnosed during her childhood. She denies any history of recent trauma, illness, or hospitalization, except for cataract surgery 2 years ago. The patient is a retired postal worker, married, and living with her husband in a senior housing condominium. She quit smoking cigarettes at age 40 and reports occasional use of alcohol (about one glass of wine weekly). She is on a DASH diet with regular exercises through a support group from her church.

Allergies

Penicillin (skin rash); no known food allergies.

Medications

- Metformin 850 mg BID.
- Hydrochlorothiazide/lisinopril 12.5 mg/20 mg QD.
- Atorvastatin 10 mg QHS.
- OTC multivitamin.

Physical Examination

- *Vitals:* T 37°C (98.6°F), P 90, R 16, BP 135/80, WT 90 kg (198.4 lb), HT 170 cm (66.9 in.), BMI 32.9.
- *General:* Well-developed and nourished White woman in no acute distress. She appears mildly anxious but A&O×4.

- *Skin, Hair, and Nails:* Skin was fair, warm, and moist with good skin turgor. No jaundice, erythema, rashes, or scales noted. There are no signs of nodularity, thickening, or pain on skin palpation. Hair and nails showed no abnormal findings.
- *Head:* She has no lesions, scaling, or scalp tenderness.
- *Eyes:* Vision is reduced bilaterally (20/30 in the OD; blurred in OS but able to count fingers at 3 feet); pupils were reactive to light. EOM are full, but patient has both temporal and nasal visual field deficits in the OS. Tonometry measuring of IOP: 17 mmHg in the OD and 12 mmHg in the OS.
- *ENT/Mouth:* Ears, nares, mouth, and throat have no abnormal findings.
- *Neck:* Supple with no cervical adenopathy or thyroid enlargement.
- *Lungs:* Respiratory rate is 16 and unlabored. Trachea is midline. She has normal anteroposterior diameter. No tenderness on palpation. Tactile fremitus and respiratory expansion are normal. The lungs are CTA. No wheezes, crackles, or rhonchi bilaterally.
- *Heart:* RRR, without murmur, gallop, or rub.
- *Peripheral Vascular:* Dorsalis pedis and posterior tibial pulses are faint (1/4).
- *Neurologic:* A&O. Most CNs are intact. Sensation and reflexes are present in all extremities.

Clinical Discussion Questions

1. What is the differential diagnosis?

2. What is the most likely diagnosis? Why?

3. Demonstrate your understanding about the pathophysiology of the most likely diagnosis.

4. Should tests/imaging studies be ordered? Which ones? Why? Think about tests/imaging beyond the primary care setting as well.

5. What are the next appropriate steps in management?

6. Review recent and credible research articles on about this diagnosis. Demonstrate your understanding of the diagnostic criteria, supplemental testing, and treatment approach. Provide references with your response.

7. What are the pertinent ICD-10 and CPT (E/M) codes for this visit? Provide a short rationale.

8. What are the appropriate patient education topics for this case?

9. If not managed appropriately, what is/are the medical/legal concern(s) that may arise?

10. Think about interprofessional collaboration for this case. Provide a list of specialties or other disciplines and indicate what contribution these professionals might make to managing the patient.

Bedside Manner Question

11. What would your communication style/approach be with this patient?

Answers available at courseconnect.springerpub.com.

CASE 20

SORE THROAT, FEVER, AND CHILLS, ADULT MALE

Chief Complaint

"Sore throat, fever, and chills."

History of Present Illness

A 25-year-old man with a history of asthma and DM presents as a new patient with a 4-day history of a sore throat that had worsened overnight. His throat initially started hurting 4 to 5 days ago; however, he now has associated subjective fever, chills, and pain upon swallowing. The pain is burning, constant, rated 8/10, and radiates to his left ear. He has been taking ibuprofen the last 4 days without significant relief. The patient has had sore throats prior to this episode, but he has "never had pain like this before." Previous episodes typically occurred with symptoms of a "cold" and lasted 1 to 2 days. He is able to tolerate soft foods and liquids. He is accompanied today by his father.

Review of Systems

The patient's ROS is positive for fever, chills, odynophagia, trismus, and otalgia. His ROS is negative for malaise, fatigue, nausea, vomiting, cough, SOB, hemoptysis, abdominal pain, neck pain, and rash.

Relevant History

The patient's relevant history is positive for T2DM and asthma, both well controlled. He is married and has one daughter. He denies tobacco use, drinks "a few" beers on the weekend, smokes marijuana on occasion, and denies other recreational drugs. His father is well, with chronic, uncomplicated DM and HTN. His mother is alive and well with chronic HTN complicated by CKD.

Allergies

No known drug allergies; no known food allergies.

Medications

- Albuterol inhaler two puffs inhaled, Q4h to Q6h PRN.
- Metformin 500 mg PO BID.

Physical Examination

- *Vitals:* T 38.1°C (100.5°F), P 103, R 18, BP 132/78, SpO_2 99%, WT 90.72 kg (200 lb), HT 182.88 cm (72 in.), BMI 27.12.
- *General:* Ill-appearing male sitting on the bed, in mild distress related to pain. Patient is speaking in short sentences, and his voice is muffled and low pitch in quality.
- *Psychiatric:* Cooperative, mildly anxious secondary to pain.
- *Skin, Hair, and Nails:* No rashes or abnormal pigmentation noted. No abnormal findings with hair or nails.
- *Head:* Atraumatic, normocephalic.
- *Eyes:* Conjunctiva pink and moist, PERRLA, EOMI.

- *ENT/Mouth:* Bilateral TM intact, pearly gray in color, cone of light noted, serous fluid appreciated on the left; no erythema or exudates noted. Mucosa pink and moist; no lesions, swelling, or drainage noted in nose. Difficulty opening his mouth. Buccal mucosa slightly dry; posterior pharynx is erythematous; mild white tonsillar exudate bilateral, (2+) tonsillar enlargement on the right, (3+) tonsillar enlargement on the left, and deviation of the uvula toward the right noted.
- *Neck:* Supple, no bruits appreciated, trachea midline, no thyromegaly appreciated, lymphadenopathy noted with tender to palpation at site of the left submandibular region and along the left superficial cervical chain.
- *Lungs:* Normal anteroposterior diameter; nonlabored breathing; symmetric chest wall expansion; no chest wall tenderness to palpation; breath sounds CTA bilaterally, without wheezing, rales, or rhonchi.
- *Heart:* RRR, S1 and S2 present (normal); no murmurs, rubs, or gallops.
- *Abdomen:* Nondistended, positive BS, soft, nontender; no masses or splenomegaly appreciated.
- *Neurologic:* A&O×3. CN II to XII grossly intact.

CLINICAL DISCUSSION QUESTIONS

1. What is the differential diagnosis?

2. What is the most likely diagnosis? Why?

3. Demonstrate your understanding about the pathophysiology of the most likely diagnosis.

4. Should tests/imaging studies be ordered? Which ones? Why? Think about tests/imaging beyond the primary care setting as well.

5. What are the next appropriate steps in management?

6. What are the risk factors and predictors for hospitalization for the diagnosis? Provide references for your response.

7. What are the pertinent ICD-10 and CPT (E/M) codes for this visit? Provide a short rationale.

8. What is the appropriate patient education topic for this case?

9. If not managed appropriately, what is/are the medical/legal concern(s) that may arise?

10. Think about interprofessional collaboration for this case. Provide a list of specialties or other disciplines and indicate what contribution these professionals might make to managing the patient.

BEDSIDE MANNER QUESTIONS

11. What would your communication style/approach be with this patient and his father?

12. If a patient and his father are distressed by the diagnosis, what might offer support?

Answers available at courseconnect.springerpub.com.

CASE 21

HEART PALPITATIONS, ADULT FEMALE

Chief Complaint

"Heart palpitations."

History of Present Illness

A 64-year-old woman presents to her regular PCP complaining of chest palpitations. She was watching TV and suddenly her heart started racing and pounding. She became lightheaded and felt a bit better after a while. She reports she hears her heart beating when lying down. She is concerned and now presents for evaluation. She reports having mild palpitations in the past but nothing like this. She has a history of atrial fibrillation and was taken off her blood thinners by her urologist and oncologist. She was diagnosed with kidney cancer 5 months ago and is now 4 months post right nephrectomy. She denies any chest pain or syncope. She reports she never refilled her previous medication and she did not follow up with her PCP post-surgery.

Review of Systems

The patient's ROS is positive for chest palpitations, generalized weakness, and SOB. Her ROS is negative for weight loss or gain, fever, chills, vomiting, diarrhea, constipation, and chest pain.

Relevant History

This patient has a history of HTN, renal cancer, CAD, GERD, and a systolic murmur. She also has a new lung lesion. Her surgical history is positive for a nephrectomy 4 months ago. The patient is a widow and lives with her only child, an unmarried son. She denies tobacco use, alcohol use, or any illicit drug use. She has a family history of CAD, HTN, and T2DM but no family history of cancer.

Allergies

No known drug allergies; no known food allergies.

Medications

- Diltiazem 180 mg PO QD (empty pill bottle).
- Lisinopril 20 mg PO QD.
- Metoprolol succinate 50 mg QD (empty pill bottle).
- Low-dose aspirin 81 mg PO QD.

Physical Examination

- *Vitals:* T 36.8°C (98.3°F), P 130, R 18, BP 110/74, WT 80.7 kg (178 lb), HT 160 cm (63 in.), BMI 31.5.
- *General:* Lethargic but not in acute distress.
- *Psychiatric:* Smiles; is cooperative and answers all questions appropriately though slightly slow to respond, but states this is her baseline after the nephrectomy and her surgeon said it is to be expected.
- *Lungs:* Nonlabored, chest rise symmetrical, lungs CTA bilaterally.

- *Heart:* Irregular rhythm and rapid heart rate, systolic murmur right sternal border grade 3/6.
- *Neurologic:* Alert and awake (GCS = 15), but delayed verbal response; motor and sensory is intact; deep tendon reflex 2+ bilaterally; Romberg is negative.

Clinical Discussion Questions

1. What is the differential diagnosis?

2. What is the most likely diagnosis? Why?

3. Demonstrate your understanding about the pathophysiology of the most likely diagnosis.

4. Should tests/imaging studies be ordered? Which ones? Why? Think about tests/imaging beyond the primary care setting as well.

5. What are the next appropriate steps in management?

6. What are the prevalence, incidence, and complications of the diagnosis? Provide references for your responses.

7. What are the pertinent ICD-10 and CPT (E/M) codes for this visit? Provide a short rationale.

8. What is the appropriate patient education topic for this case?

9. If not managed appropriately, what is/are the medical/legal concern(s) that may arise?

10. Think about interprofessional collaboration for this case. Provide a list of specialties or other disciplines and indicate what contribution these professionals might make to managing the patient.

BEDSIDE MANNER QUESTION

11. What would your communication style/approach be with this patient?

Answers available at courseconnect.springerpub.com.

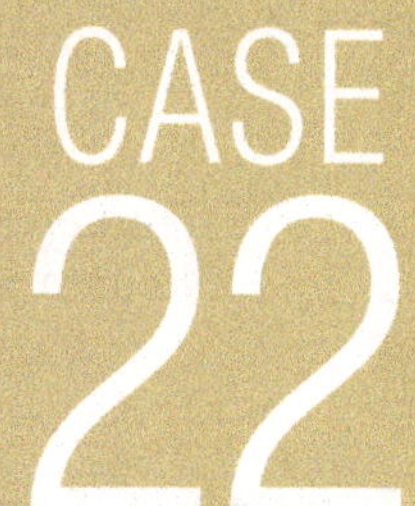

NIPPLE PAIN, ADULT FEMALE

Chief Complaint

"Nipple pain."

History of Present Illness

A 34-year-old White woman presents to her PCP with a 3-day history of pain in her right nipple. She presents to the appointment alone and is a good historian. She is married, the mother of two children ages 3 years and 9 months, and is a part-time loan officer at a local bank. She is currently breastfeeding and began to wean her youngest about 1 week ago. She generally breastfeeds at night and pumps for daytime feedings. Three days ago, she experienced sharp shooting pains in the right nipple with some radiation to the right axilla. She described the pain as 6/10 on a 0-to-10 pain scale. She has tried white willow bark, cool compresses, and breast massage for letdown of milk without any success. Today, she presents with continued complaints of right nipple pain, some malaise, headache, and "not feeling well."

Review of Systems

The patient's ROS is positive for breast pain with radiation, low-grade fever, and malaise. Her ROS is negative for breast lump, erythema, or nipple discharge, sleep disturbance, irritability or sadness, numbness, or tingling.

Relevant History

The patient is generally healthy with no major health problems. Her obstetric history is G2 P2 NSVD, with both deliveries born at home at term with midwife assistance. No postpartum difficulties. Both children were breastfed.

Allergies

No known drug allergies; no known food allergies.

Medications

None.

Physical Examination

- *Vitals:* T 37.9°C (100.2°F), P 76, R 20, BP 118/64, WT 55.3 kg (122 lb), HT 165.1 cm (65 in.), BMI 20.5.
- *General:* In mild discomfort. Appears fatigued.
- *Psychiatric:* Affect is normal and appropriate.
- *Lungs:* Respirations even and unlabored, clear bilaterally.
- *Heart:* Normal S1, S2; without rubs, murmurs, or gallops.
- *Right Breast:* Full without engorgement. Mild pain to palpation of nipple radiating to 3 o'clock location and right axilla. Mild breast erythema noted. No nipple discharge without stimulation; upon stimulation able to obtain specimen.

- *Musculoskeletal:* Motor 5/5 proximal and distal UEs, including shoulders. DTRs 2+ and symmetrical of knees, brachioradialis, and biceps tendons. BL upper grips equal and strong. No pain with ROM.
- *Neurologic:* A&O×3, CN II to XII grossly intact.

CLINICAL DISCUSSION QUESTIONS

1. What is the differential diagnosis?

2. What is the most likely diagnosis? Why?

3. Demonstrate your understanding about the pathophysiology of the most likely diagnosis.

4. Should tests/imaging studies be ordered? Which ones? Why? Think about tests/imaging beyond the primary care setting as well.

5. What are the next appropriate steps in management?

6. What are the causing pathogens and treatment options for this diagnosis? Provide references for your response.

7. What are the pertinent ICD-10 and CPT (E/M) codes for this visit? Provide a short rationale.

8. What is the appropriate patient education topic for this case?

9. If not managed appropriately, what is/are the medical/legal concern(s) that may arise?

10. Think about interprofessional collaboration for this case. Provide a list of specialties or other disciplines and indicate what contribution these professionals might make to managing the patient.

BEDSIDE MANNER QUESTION

11. What would your communication style/approach be with this patient?

Answers available at courseconnect.springerpub.com.

CASE 23

RECURRENT PAIN AND REDNESS IN LEFT FOOT, ADULT FEMALE

Chief Complaint

"Recurrent pain and redness in left foot."

History of Present Illness

A 36-year-old woman presents to her PCP with increased pain in her left foot. The pain has been present for the past 3 months but has gotten worse over the past week. She also complains of an intermittent low-grade fever and chills. Her fever comes and goes but is present mainly at night. She states that 6 months ago, she had a similar episode and was seen at an urgent care, where antibiotics were prescribed and her pain subsided. Today, she complains the pain has been gradually increasing and her lower left leg is warm to touch and red. The pain and swelling increase with activity. Elevating and resting the foot decreases the pain and swelling but her symptoms return as soon as she resumes activity. She denies any injury or trauma to her left leg or foot.

Review of Systems

The patient's ROS is positive for a low-grade fever, chills, left foot swelling, redness, and pain to the left foot. The patient reported malaise and fatigue and pain and redness to the left foot. Her ROS is negative for nausea, vomiting, decreased appetite, chest pain, or SOB. She denies hip or knee pain or any recent injury or trauma.

Relevant History

The patient has T2DM and HTN (age 28). Six months ago, she developed a wound over the left ankle and foot that is now closed. The patient is a smoker of one pack of cigarettes/day. She is single and lives alone with her two dogs and three cats. Her family history includes DM and HTN.

Allergies

No known drug allergies; no known food allergies.

Medications

- Metformin 1,000 mg BID.
- Enalapril 10 mg QD.

Physical Examination

- *Vitals:* T 38.1°C (100.6°F), P 82, R 20, BP 128/82, WT 68 kg (150 lb), HT 165 cm (65 in.), BMI 24.2.
- *General:* Alert and cooperative. Sitting comfortably on the exam table. Does not have a toxic or distressed appearance. Well hydrated, well nourished.
- *Skin, Hair, and Nails:* Skin warm and dry. Rest of the exam within normal findings.
- *Neck:* Supple with FROM and no lymphadenopathy present.
- *Lungs:* CTA bilaterally. No rales or rhonchi present.
- *Heart:* RRR. Normal S2.

- *Musculoskeletal:* At the left ankle and foot, diffuse blanching erythema and trace nonpitting edema noted. At the dorsum of the left foot and anterolateral aspect of the talofibular joint, there is a 3 × 3 cm^2 area of erythema and warmth, tender to palpation. FROM to ankle.
- *Neurologic:* Left foot with normal sensation and 2+ pedal pulse to posterior tibia and dorsalis pedis. No drop foot present.

Clinical Discussion Questions

1. What is the differential diagnosis?

2. What is the most likely diagnosis? Why?

3. Demonstrate your understanding about the pathophysiology of the most likely diagnosis.

4. Should tests/imaging studies be ordered? Which ones? Why? Think about tests/imaging beyond the primary care setting as well.

5. What are the next appropriate steps in management?

6. What is the treatment approach for this diagnosis? Provide references for your response.

7. What are the pertinent ICD-10 and CPT (E/M) codes for this visit? Provide a short rationale.

8. What is the appropriate patient education topic for this case?

9. If not managed appropriately, what is/are the medical/legal concern(s) that may arise?

10. Think about interprofessional collaboration for this case. Provide a list of specialties or other disciplines and indicate what contribution these professionals might make to managing the patient.

BEDSIDE MANNER QUESTION

11. What would your communication style/approach be with this patient?

Answers available at courseconnect.springerpub.com.

CASE 24

MUSCLE AND JOINT PAIN, ADULT FEMALE

Chief Complaint

"Muscle and joint pain."

History of Present Illness

A 45-year-old woman presents to her PCP with muscle and joint pain. She complains of fatigue, headache, neck stiffness, and poor appetite. She returned to California last night from Rhode Island, where she had been on a summer camping trip with several close friends. She camped for 2 days at the beginning of her 10-day trip. She denies fever, chills, nausea, vomiting, constipation, abdominal pain, cough, runny nose, sore throat, ear pain, nasal congestion, rash, dysuria, urinary urgency, SOB, or chest pain. Her husband camped with her. She does not recall seeing any ticks while camping. She denies having a tick bite. However, she recalls one of her friends screamed that she saw a tick on her lower leg. When asked for more information about her husband, she states he is doing well but just tired from the long trip. When asked if he had seen any ticks during the camping, she states, "He didn't mention anything like that." When asked if her husband has any rash, she states, "Yes. He noticed ringworm this morning and applied some topical cream." She states her husband gets ringworm occasionally from their dog.

Review of Systems

The patient's ROS is positive for muscle pain, joint pain, neck stiffness, and anorexia. She reports fatigue and headache. Her ROS is negative for fever, chills, nausea, vomiting, constipation, abdominal pain, cough, runny nose, sore throat, ear pain, nasal congestion, rash, dysuria, urinary urgency, SOB, and chest pain.

Relevant History

The patient's history is significant for hypothyroidism (onset age 30), benign HTN (onset age 35), hypercholesteremia (onset age 30), and obesity. She had two Cesarean sections. She has had no other surgeries. Her social history includes traveling with her husband. She has been working as a referral clerk for a healthcare clinic. She has one sister and one brother. She has been sexually active (no protection) since age 20 with her husband and they are in a monogamous relationship. Her family history includes DM, MI, and CAD in her father and breast cancer, hypothyroidism, and DM in her mother. Her family history is negative for autoimmune disease.

Allergies

No known drug allergies; no known food allergies.

Medications

- Levothyroxine 50 mcg QD.
- Hydrochlorothiazide/lisinopril 12.5 mg/10 mg QD.
- Atorvastatin 20 mg QD.

PHYSICAL EXAMINATION

- *Vitals:* T 37.2°C (99.0°F), P 78, R 18, BP 130/86, HT 162.6 cm (64 in.), WT 73.9 kg (163 lb), BMI 28.
- *General:* No acute distress, communicates well, afebrile.
- *Psychiatric:* Appropriate mood and affect.
- *Skin, Hair, and Nails:* No skin rash or lesion appreciated. No abnormal findings with hair or nails.
- *Eyes:* Conjunctiva and sclera clear, no injection or exudate.
- *ENT/Mouth:* Ear canals clear, TMs pearly gray, intact with normal light reflex. No nasal deformity, pharynx without erythema or exudate.
- *Lungs:* CTA, good air movements throughout.
- *Heart:* RRR, no murmurs, radial and femoral pulses strong and equal.
- *Abdomen:* Soft, nontender, not distended.
- *Lymphatic:* Palpable lymph nodes on cervical, axillary (BL), and inguinal (BL).
- *Musculoskeletal:* Muscle strength appropriate and equal bilaterally, full range of active and passive motion; muscle tenderness noted; generalized.
- *Neurologic:* A&O×3, CN II to XII intact.

CLINICAL DISCUSSION QUESTIONS

1. What is the differential diagnosis?

___

___

___

___

2. What is the most likely diagnosis? Why?

___

___

___

___

3. Demonstrate your understanding about the pathophysiology of the most likely diagnosis.

___

___

___

___

4. Should tests/imaging studies be ordered? Which ones? Why? Think about tests/imaging beyond the primary care setting as well.

5. What are the next appropriate steps in management?

6. Review a reliable, recent source and discuss screening labs, diagnosis criteria, and treatment plans for the diagnosis. Provide references for your responses.

7. What are the pertinent ICD-10 and CPT (E/M) codes for this visit? Provide a short rationale.

8. What is the appropriate patient education topic for this case?

9. If not managed appropriately, what is/are the medical/legal concern(s) that may arise?

10. Think about interprofessional collaboration for this case. Provide a list of specialties or other disciplines and indicate what contribution these professionals might make to managing the patient.

BEDSIDE MANNER QUESTION

11. What would your communication style/approach be with this patient?

Answers available at courseconnect.springerpub.com.

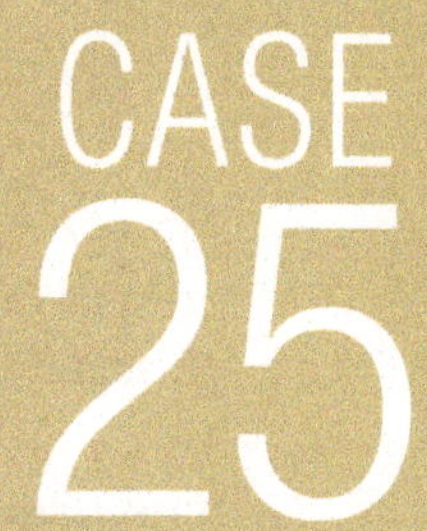

CASE 25

DOUBLE VISION, ADULT FEMALE

Chief Complaint

"Double vision and eye drooping."

History of Present Illness

A 28-year-old woman presents to the primary care clinic for evaluation of sudden-onset, painless double vision and a drooping right eyelid for 7 days. The symptoms began upon awakening 7 days ago and remain constant throughout the day, with nothing seeming to alleviate them. She has found driving and reading challenging—both essential tasks for her job. Her double vision worsens when she gazes to the right. She describes her vision as seeing objects appearing "one on top of the other." She has had no recent headaches, head trauma, loss of consciousness, or weakness. She has had no change in speech, memory, or mental status.

Review of Systems

The patient's ROS is positive for double vision and drooping right eyelid. ROS is negative for head trauma, headaches, changes in balance or coordination, numbness, tingling, weakness in the extremity, changes in speech or hearing, syncope, lightheadedness, dizziness, loss of consciousness, tinnitus, or hyperacusis. The patient also denies depression, changes in weight or appetite, fatigue, difficulty sleeping, anxiety, chest pain, palpitations, or difficulty breathing.

Relevant History

The patient's medical history shows no significant childhood diagnoses, no significant adult diagnoses, and no history of surgery.

The patient's social history shows no current or previous smoking or tobacco use, and no current or previous illicit drug use. The patient consumes 6 alcoholic drinks per week (red wine, beer, mixed drinks), and she does not drink more than 1 drink per day. This has been her pattern for 5 to 6 years. She lives alone, exercises 4 times per week (60 minutes running and 30 minutes resistance training), and has been sexually active with 3 male partners in the last year with barrier method contraception used each time.

The patient's family history is noncontributory; her mother is alive (age 53) with no health problems; her father (age 57) has had T2DM for 6 years. She has no family history of known ophthalmologic, endocrine, or neurologic disorders.

Allergies

Penicillin (rash); no known food allergies.

Medications

Daily multivitamin.

Physical Examination

- *Vitals*: T 37°C (98.6°F), P 62, R 12, BP 110/62, HT 165.1 cm (65 in.), WT 65.31 kg (144 lb), BMI 24.0.
- *General:* Well-appearing 28-year-old female in no acute distress.
- *Psychiatric:* Cooperative with exam, clean, A&O×3, affect full and appropriate.

- *Skin, Hair, and Nails:* Skin intact without sloughing or dry patches; hair full without thinning.
- *EENT/Mouth:* Drooping upper lid OD. Gaze turned laterally and inferiorly, and lid lag present OD. EOMs restricted in all directions except for laterally OD. EOMI in OS. Pupil enlarged OD > OS. Pupil OD unresponsive to light; left pupil constricts normally.
- *Musculoskeletal:* FROM in the cervical spine; negative tenderness to palpation of paracervical musculature.
- *Neurologic:* DTRs 2+ equal and symmetrical in BL upper and lower extremities. Tone within normal limits with passive motion in BL upper and lower extremities. Strength 5/5 in BL upper and lower extremities. Negative Babinski, negative clonus. Negative Kerning, negative Brudzinski.

CLINICAL DISCUSSION QUESTIONS

1. What is the differential diagnosis?

____

____

____

____

2. What is the most likely diagnosis? Why?

____

____

____

____

3. Demonstrate your understanding about the pathophysiology of the most likely diagnosis.

____

____

____

____

4. Should tests/imaging studies be ordered? Which ones? Why? Think about tests/imaging beyond the primary care setting as well.

____

____

____

____

5. What are the next appropriate steps in management?

6. What are the treatment options for this diagnosis? Provide references for your response.

7. What are the pertinent ICD-10 and CPT (E/M) codes for this visit? Provide a short rationale.

8. What is the appropriate patient education topic for this case?

9. If not managed appropriately, what is/are the medical/legal concern(s) that may arise?

10. Think about interprofessional collaboration for this case. Provide a list of specialties or other disciplines and indicate what contribution these professionals might make to managing the patient.

BEDSIDE MANNER QUESTION

11. How would you communicate your likely diagnosis to the patient?

____

____

____

____

Answers available at courseconnect.springerpub.com.

CASE 26

PAINLESS ANAL BUMPS, ADULT TRANSGENDER MALE

Chief Complaint

"Painless anal bumps."

History of Present Illness

A 23-year-old transgender man presents to a new PCP with a several-month history of painless lesions around his anal area. He first noticed them while showering; they felt like little skin tags and were painless. Early on, he could only feel two or three. He states those are larger now, and more have emerged around the anus. He states they sometimes bleed after a bowel movement. He is sexually active with a self-identified gender-nonconforming partner with male genitalia, and they engage in both vaginal and anal sex where the patient is the receptive partner. He denies any other history of STIs and gets regular HIV testing, and the last routine screens for HIV and STI testing at the local health department were negative.

The patient did see a local urgent care provider last week about his complaints. The clinician told him that they looked like skin tags but might be warts, and if he waited, they should go away on their own. They have not, and this is why he has come to today's appointment.

Review of Systems

The patient's ROS is negative for any similar skin rashes on other areas of the body. He denies any vaginal or anal discharge or bleeding. He also denies any symptoms of fever, chills, changes in bowel habits, chest pain, abdominal pain, SOB, or any constitutional symptoms.

Relevant History

The patient's medical history is significant for elevated BP as told to him by a previous PCP, but he has never been diagnosed with HTN and he takes no BP medications. His surgical history is significant for a tonsillectomy at age 18. He lives with his partner; they have been together for 2 years, and he denies other sexual partners. He states he has all his required vaccinations but does not remember if he had the HPV vaccine. He was asked to leave his parents' house at 19 when he embraced his transgender identity and has not spoken with them since; they have all his childhood medical and vaccination records. His mental health is good. He sees a therapist regularly and has never been diagnosed with any formal psychologic diagnoses.

He began his transition as a young teenager, but he only began taking hormones 3 years ago when he became comfortable sharing his identity with his medical provider. He reports no interest in a mastectomy as part of his gender confirmation at this point. He prefers to "go with the hormones" first before pursuing surgical interventions as well. He states that he has not had a full pelvic exam in years since his gender confirmation. Because none of his previous providers suggested he have one, he thought it was fine to just skip it.

He only takes injectable testosterone at this time, which he administers himself or, sometimes, his partner administers for him. His testosterone levels have ranged in the mid-400s, which he is happy with, and he has been pleased with facial hair growth, a deeper voice, and a notable increase in muscle mass. He stopped menstruating 2 years ago.

Allergies

No known drug allergies; no known food allergies.

MEDICATIONS

Testosterone 200 mg IM every 2 weeks (self-administered or administered by his partner).

PHYSICAL EXAMINATION

- *Vitals:* T 37.1°C (98.8°F), P 77, R 16, BP 128/84, WT 85.3 kg (188 lb), HT 177.8 cm (70 in.), BMI 27.
- *General:* Thin male in no apparent distress.
- *Genital/Rectal:* Pelvic exam reveals unremarkable vaginal anatomy, no lesions or rashes noted, no cervical lesions or discharge noted. Rectal exam reveals multiple (>5) verruca-appearing lesions varying from 1 to 3 cm. No tenderness to palpation noted; no evidence of external bleeding. All lesions are immediately at the anal verge or immediately surrounding it, without evidence of outlet obstruction.

CLINICAL DISCUSSION QUESTIONS

1. What is the differential diagnosis?

2. What is the most likely diagnosis? Why?

3. Demonstrate your understanding about the pathophysiology of the most likely diagnosis.

4. Should tests/imaging studies be ordered? Which ones? Why? Think about tests/imaging beyond the primary care setting as well.

5. What are the next appropriate steps in management?

6. Review a reliable, recent source and demonstrate an understanding of the prevalence, prevention, and treatments. Provide references for your responses.

7. What are the pertinent ICD-10 and CPT (E/M) codes for this visit? Provide a short rationale.

8. What is the appropriate patient education topic for this case?

9. If not managed appropriately, what is/are the medical/legal concern(s) that may arise?

10. Think about interprofessional collaboration for this case. Provide a list of specialties or other disciplines and indicate what contribution these professionals might make to managing the patient.

Bedside Manner Questions

11. What would your communication style/approach be with this patient?

12. If a patient is distressed by the diagnosis, what might offer support?

Answers available at courseconnect.springerpub.com.

CASE 27

FATIGUE AND DECREASED LIBIDO, ADULT MALE

Chief Complaint

"Fatigue and decreased libido."

History of Present Illness

A 35-year-old man with a history of HTN and obesity presents to his PCP with a complaint of fatigue. He works as an accountant and is married with three children. The patient reports that over the last year, he has gained weight, been tired, and is less motivated to work. He also had decreased libido that is causing marital stress. He recalls that 5 years ago, he was much more active, going to the gym and running regularly, he but now he does not have the energy or the motivation to exercise. He has noticed a steady weight gain over the years. He has gained about 75 lb over the last 6 years. When asked about his mood, he describes being depressed, and he has not been going out with his friends or his family. He says he sometimes sleeps until someone wakes him up or he is "forced" to get up.

Review of Systems

The patient's ROS is positive for fatigue, weight gain, decreased libido, lack of motivation, and distraction at work with difficulty concentrating. His ROS is negative for dry hair or nails, constipation, palpitations, SOB, or chills.

Relevant History

The patient's history is significant for HTN and obesity that developed over the last 3 years. The patient denies any surgeries and denies any family history of cancer or thyroid disease. He does report his mother has HTN. He denies drugs and tobacco. He drinks two to three beers once or twice a month.

Allergies

No known drug allergies; no known food allergies.

Medications

Lisinopril 5 mg QD.

Physical Examination

- *Vitals:* T 36.5°C (97.8°F), R 20, P 72, BP 134/79, HT 177.8 cm (70 in.), WT 110.7 kg (244 lb), BMI 35.
- *General:* No acute distress, obese.
- *Psychiatric:* Low affect.
- *Skin, Hair, and Nails:* Normal turgor, no rash or dryness noted, no sign of hair loss.
- *ENT /Mouth:* Moist mucosa.
- *Lungs:* CTA bilaterally.
- *Breasts:* Gynecomastia BL, no masses.
- *Heart:* RRR, no murmur.
- *Abdomen:* Nondistended, nontender, BS present.

- *Genital/Rectal:* Testicles small bilaterally, length of testes measures approximately 3 cm bilaterally. No masses, no tenderness. No hernias. Rectal exam deferred.
- *Neurologic:* No focal deficits.

CLINICAL DISCUSSION QUESTIONS

1. What is the differential diagnosis?

2. What is the most likely diagnosis? Why?

3. Demonstrate your understanding about the pathophysiology of the most likely diagnosis.

4. Should tests/imaging studies be ordered? Which ones? Why? Think about tests/imaging beyond the primary care setting as well.

5. What are the next appropriate steps in management?

6. Review a reliable, recent source and discuss the treatment approach and contributing factors of the diagnosis. Provide references for your responses.

7. What are the pertinent ICD-10 and CPT (E/M) codes for this visit? Provide a short rationale.

8. What is the appropriate patient education topic for this case?

9. If not managed appropriately, what is/are the medical/legal concern(s) that may arise?

10. Think about interprofessional collaboration for this case. Provide a list of specialties or other disciplines and indicate what contribution these professionals might make to managing the patient.

Bedside Manner Questions

11. What would your communication style/approach be with this patient?

12. If a patient is distressed by the diagnosis, what might offer support?

____

____

____

____

Answers available at courseconnect.springerpub.com.

CASE 28

FEVER AND BODY ACHES, ADULT MALE

Chief Complaint

"Fever and body aches."

History of Present Illness

A 39-year-old male shipbuilder reports to his PCP's office in late February 2020 with a 24-hour history of fever and generalized body aches. The fever came on suddenly while he was at work yesterday, and he worked through the remaining 3 hours of his shift before going home. He does not own a thermometer so he did not check his temperature at home. He admits to feeling sluggish over the same period. The achiness is most pronounced in his back and shoulders and he rates it as 7/10 on a pain scale. Since the onset of his symptoms, the patient admits to chills, dry cough, headache, and runny nose. He has not taken anything OTC to alleviate his symptoms. He has two children in grade school who have been sick recently but states that neither missed school because they never ran a fever. The patient is up to date on all vaccinations except annual influenza. He states that after getting the flu shot several years ago, he contracted the flu a few days after and has not been vaccinated since.

Review of Systems

The patient's ROS is positive for generalized achiness, fever, chills, fatigue, headache, rhinorrhea, dry cough, and decrease in appetite. The patient denied ear pain, sore throat, wheezing, SOB, sinus congestion, eye pain or itching, diarrhea, nausea or vomiting, or chest pain.

Relevant History

The patient has a medical history of HTN treated with lisinopril and hydrochlorothiazide. He works in a local shipyard as a welder. He is married with two children. There are no pets in the home. He does not regularly "go to the doctor" but comes to the office at least annually for his employee physical. He has smoked about 1 pack per day for the last 19 years, drinks one to two beers on the weekend, and denies the use of street drugs. His family history is unknown as he was adopted.

Allergies

No known drug allergies; no known food allergies.

Medications

Lisinopril/hydrochlorothiazide 20 mg/12.5 mg PO QD.

Physical Examination

- *Vitals:* T 39.5°C (103.1°F), P 104, R 19, BP 130/85, HT 187.96 cm (74 in.), WT 113.85 kg (251 lb), BMI 32.
- *General:* Well developed, obese, in no acute distress but appears to be ill.
- *Psychiatric:* Normal mood and affect.
- *ENT/Mouth:* TMs pearly gray without effusion or bulging; inferior turbinates swollen, boggy, and erythematous; oropharynx without exudates but injection is present. There is no tonsillar hypertrophy. Mildly tender anterior cervical lymphadenopathy bilaterally.
- *Heart:* Regular rhythm; mild tachycardia present; no murmurs, rubs, or gallops.
- *Lungs:* CTA bilaterally.

Clinical Discussion Questions

1. What is the differential diagnosis?

2. What is the most likely diagnosis? Why?

3. Demonstrate your understanding about the pathophysiology of the most likely diagnosis.

4. Should tests/imaging studies be ordered? Which ones? Why? Think about tests/imaging beyond the primary care setting as well.

5. What are the next appropriate steps in management?

6. What are the diagnostic criteria, treatments, and prevention for this diagnosis? Provide reference(s) for your responses.

7. What are the pertinent ICD-10 and CPT (E/M) codes for this visit? Provide a short rationale.

8. What is the appropriate patient education topic for this case?

9. If not managed appropriately, what is/are the medical/legal concern(s) that may arise?

10. Think about interprofessional collaboration for this case. Provide a list of specialties or other disciplines and indicate what contribution these professionals might make to managing the patient.

BEDSIDE MANNER QUESTIONS

11. What would your communication style/approach be with this patient?

12. If a patient is distressed by the diagnosis, what might offer support?

Answers available at courseconnect.springerpub.com.

EYE PAIN AND BLURRY VISION, ADULT FEMALE

CASE 29

Chief Complaint

"Eye pain and blurry vision after skiing."

History of Present Illness

A 42-year-old White woman presents to a primary care clinic in Colorado as a walk-inpatient with a painful OS and associated blurred vision. She is currently on vacation (normally lives on the East Coast). Patient has been skiing all day today, on a bright sunny day at high altitude (elevation of 10,000 feet). She lost her goggles on the mountain this morning, so she was not able to wear them. She states her OS has been tearing, pink, and irritated, with a "gritty" sensation since 11:00 AM this morning. Her OS started hurting around 4:00 PM, with pain rated at 5 out of 10. She also reports mild photophobia, as well as slightly blurred vision which clears when she wipes away tears. Patient also reports a "sunburn" on exposed facial skin.

She notes that her OD is not painful or irritated, and her vision is normal. She denies any speech/motor deficits, known foreign bodies, discharge from the eyes, sick contacts, or any direct trauma to either eye. She does not wear contact lenses, nor does she wear glasses. She denies any history of immunodeficiency or recent international travel.

Review of Systems

The patient's ROS is positive for an irritated, painful OS with associated tearing, blurry vision, photophobia, and redness. Her ROS is negative for fever, chills, fatigue, eyelid swelling, eyelid redness, recent illness, breaks in skin, rashes, or bites.

Relevant History

The patient reports being healthy and having no significant medical issues nor surgeries. She is in a monogamous marriage with a male partner. She has two school-aged children, delivered vaginally at term. She has routine wellness visits, and her immunizations are up to date. Family history is not significant.

Allergies

No known drug allergies; no known food allergies.

Medications

None.

Physical Examination

- *Vitals:* T 37.1°C (98.7°F), P 66, R 16, BP 112/72, HT 162.5 cm (64 in.), WT 56.3 kg (124 lb), BMI 21.3.
- *General:* Well-appearing 42-year-old woman in no acute distress.
- *Psychiatric:* Affect and mood are appropriate to setting.
- *Skin, Hair, and Nails:* No rashes noted; mild erythema noted to cheeks, nose, and lips.
- *Head:* No evidence of trauma, bleeding, or bruising.

- *Eyes:* EOMI, PERRLA. Penlight exam demonstrates no evidence of globe rupture, no blood or white cells noted in anterior chamber, corneal clear bilaterally, conjunctivae mildly injected on the right. No fluorescein uptake or obvious foreign body noted. No swelling around either eye. No pain with EOMs.
- *Visual Acuity (Snellen Chart):*
  - OD 20/20
  - OS 20/40
  - OU 20/30
  - Tonometry shows IOP of 14 OD and 18 OS.
- *Neurologic:* A&O×3, gait intact.

Clinical Discussion Questions

1. What is the differential diagnosis?

2. What is the most likely diagnosis? Why?

3. Demonstrate your understanding about the pathophysiology of the most likely diagnosis.

4. Should tests/imaging studies be ordered? Which ones? Why? Think about tests/imaging beyond the primary care setting as well.

5. What are the next appropriate steps in management?

6. Review a reliable, recent reference regarding risk factors and treatment approaches for this diagnosis. Provide references for your response.

7. What are the pertinent ICD-10 and CPT (E/M) codes for this visit? Provide a short rationale.

8. What are appropriate patient education topics for this case?

9. If not managed appropriately, what is/are the medical/legal concern(s) that may arise?

10. Think about interprofessional collaboration for this case. Provide a list of specialties or other disciplines and indicate what contribution these professionals might make to managing the patient.

BEDSIDE MANNER QUESTION

11. What would your communication style/approach be with this patient?

____

____

____

____

Answers available at courseconnect.springerpub.com.

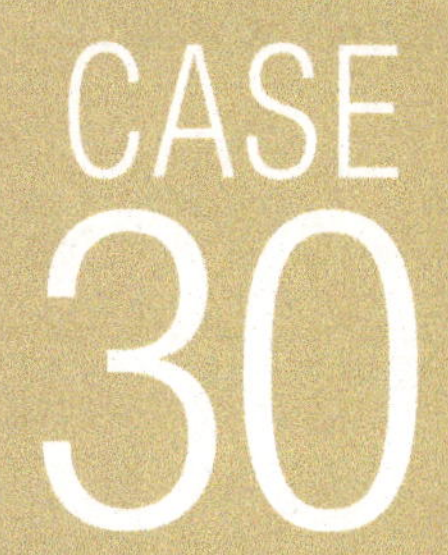

CHEST PAIN, ADULT FEMALE

Chief Complaint

"Chest pain."

History of Present Illness

A 28-year-old White woman who is a military spouse presents after a visit to an ED for recurrent episodes of chest pain. Approximately 1 year ago, she began waking abruptly at night feeling "like I'm going to die," with trembling, SOB, racing pulse, and chest discomfort lasting for 10 to 15 minutes. Her chest discomfort is described as diffuse tightness, without radiation, sweating, or nausea. Episodes were somewhat relieved by getting out of bed, walking around, and opening a window for fresh air. These episodes occurred every 3 to 4 weeks, with no known triggers; they were becoming frequent and disabling as she anticipated a recurrence. In recent months, her distress had resulted in three visits to the local ED, where she was evaluated for cardiac and pulmonary disease, ruling out AMI, angina, pulmonary embolus, and hypoglycemia (EKG, cardiac enzymes, blood work, and chest X-ray were all normal). She was told, "It's in your head," and advised not to worry about a heart attack.

The patient's main concern was that she would keep having these frightening episodes and that medical professionals could not help.

Review of Systems

The patient's ROS is positive for loneliness and anxiety that began when her military husband was deployed to the Middle East. Other psychiatric symptoms are negative, including depression, suicidal ideation, and memory problems. Her ROS is negative for fever, night sweats, weight loss, loss of appetite, loss of energy, loss of concentration, lack or excessive sleep, loss of interest, skipped heart beats, extremity swelling, wheezing, cough, nocturia/orthopnea, and heartburn.

Medical History

The patient's history is negative for major illnesses or injuries. She denies psychologic or emotional trauma. Her last routine health maintenance exam was 11 months ago for well-woman visit; results were normal.

Her immunizations are up to date. She is married to an army infantry soldier who is deployed to the Middle East. They have been married 3 years and have no children. Her family lives in a different state. She denies alcohol, tobacco, or recreational drug use. She regularly walks 2 miles for exercise.

Allergies

No known drug allergies; no known food allergies.

Medications

Levonorgestrel IUD ×3 years.

Physical Examination

- *Vitals:* T 37°C (98.7°F), P 80, R 14, BP 124/80 mmHg, HT 165 cm (65 in.), WT 62.5 kg (138 lb), BMI 23, SpO_2 99%.
- *General:* Well-developed, well-nourished woman appearing stated age.

- *Psychiatric:* A&O×3, anxious appearance.
- *Neck:* No thyromegaly, nodules, bruits, or adenopathy.
- *ENT/Mouth:* Posterior pharynx unobstructed.
- *Heart:* RRR; no murmurs, gallops, rubs, clicks; PMI nondisplaced.
- *Lungs:* CTA bilaterally; no wheezes, rales, and rhonchi; symmetric expansion; no chest wall tenderness.
- *Abdomen:* BS all quadrants, soft, nontender; no hepatosplenomegaly, no masses.
- *Extremities:* Pulses 2+ and equal; no tenderness, redness, swelling, or varicosities.

CLINICAL DISCUSSION QUESTIONS

1. What is the differential diagnosis?

2. What is the most likely diagnosis? Why?

3. Demonstrate your understanding about the pathophysiology of the most likely diagnosis.

4. Should tests/imaging studies be ordered? Which ones? Why? Think about tests/imaging beyond the primary care setting as well.

5. What are the next appropriate steps in management?

6. Review recent and credible research articles about this diagnosis. Demonstrate your understanding of the prevalence specific to this patient type and treatment options for the diagnosis. Provide references.

7. What are the pertinent ICD-10 and CPT (E/M) codes for this visit? Provide a short rationale.

8. What is the appropriate patient education topic for this case?

9. If not managed appropriately, what is/are the medical/legal concern(s) that may arise?

10. Think about interprofessional collaboration for this case. Provide a list of specialties or other disciplines and indicate what contribution these professionals might make to managing the patient.

Bedside Manner Questions

11. What would your communication style/approach be with this patient?

12. If a patient was unsure if the treatment plan is effective, how would you handle her concern?

Answers available at courseconnect.springerpub.com.

CASE 31

VAGINAL ITCHING AND INCREASED DISCHARGE, ADULT FEMALE

Chief Complaint

"Vaginal itching and increased discharge."

History of Present Illness

A 26-year-old woman presents to her PCP with a 3-day history of vaginal itching and increased discharge. She has had three other experiences with similar symptoms over the last year. She has not used any OTC medications to help resolve her symptoms. She describes the discharge as "cheese-like" and states she needs to wear a menstrual pad to catch the drainage. The itchiness is constant and is not relieved by bathing or cleansing the area. She states the area feels sore and hot and like it is burning. She is sexually active with her husband but is unable to have sexual relations due to the itchiness and pain. She does not recall having taken any antibiotics recently.

Review of Systems

The patient reports increased thick, white, and clumpy discharge that resembles cottage cheese, as well as vaginal itching, burning sensation, pain, and swelling. She denies any odor to the discharge. She endorses dysuria but reports no increased urinary frequency, pelvic pressure, or hematuria. The patient is negative for fever, chills, vomiting, nausea, lower back pain, pelvic pain, SOB, or chest pain.

Relevant History

The patient's medical history is significant for asthma and allergies. She does not drink alcohol or smoke. She reports no illicit drug usage. She is married with no other sexual partners prior to her marriage. She has 2 children. Her family history is significant for HTN.

Allergies

Codeine (hives); peanut allergy.

Medications

- Cetirizine 10 mg PO QD
- Albuterol inhaler PRN

Physical Examination

- *Vitals:* T 37°C (98.6°F), P 85, R 16, BP 106/72 mmHg, WT 64.1 kg (141.3 lb), HT 162.6 cm (64 in.), BMI 24.2.
- *General:* Well developed, well nourished, A&O, and appears to be in no acute distress.
- *Lungs:* CTA and percussion without rales, rhonchi, wheezing, or diminished breath sounds.
- *Heart:* Normal S1 and S2. Rhythm is regular.
- *Abdomen:* Positive BS. Soft, nondistended, nontender. No guarding or rebound. No masses.
- *External Genitalia:* Redness, swelling, and irritation noted to the vaginal area. There is no thinning to the skin of the external genitalia. No change in skin texture. LPN chaperoned the genital and vaginal examination.

- *Vaginal Canal Examination:* Speculum inserted to visualize the vaginal canal and cervix. Noted presence of a thick, white, clumpy discharge. Walls of the vagina are red and swollen.
- *Neurologic:* CN II–XII intact. A&O×3.

CLINICAL DISCUSSION QUESTIONS

1. What is the differential diagnosis?

2. What is the most likely diagnosis? Why?

3. Demonstrate your understanding about the pathophysiology of the most likely diagnosis.

4. Should tests/imaging studies be ordered? Which ones? Why? Think about tests/imaging beyond the primary care setting as well.

5. What are the next appropriate steps in management?

6. What are the treatment options for this diagnosis? Provide references for your response.

7. What are the pertinent ICD-10 and CPT (E/M) codes for this visit? Provide a short rationale.

8. What is the appropriate patient education topic for this case?

9. If not managed appropriately, what is/are the medical/legal concern(s) that may arise?

10. Think about interprofessional collaboration for this case. Provide a list of specialties or other disciplines and indicate what contribution these professionals might make to managing the patient.

BEDSIDE MANNER QUESTION

11. What would your communication style/approach be with this patient?

Answers available at courseconnect.springerpub.com.

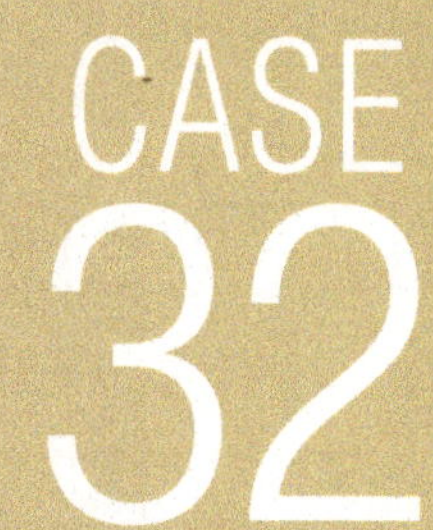

LOW PLATELETS, ADULT MALE

Chief Complaint

"Low platelets."

History of Present Illness

A new patient, age 42, is referred by his health insurance helpline to establish care and to discuss "low platelets" noted on a recent life insurance blood test. He has been without a PCP since college and has no prior labs for comparison. He feels completely well, stating he rarely gets sick and uses the local urgent care center rarely for colds and minor injuries. He denies any unusual bleeding, bruising, or skin changes. There is no known personal or family history of blood or liver disorders.

Review of Systems

The patient's ROS is negative for fever, chills, weight loss, or fatigue. He has no nasal congestion, earache, or sore throat. He reports no vision changes, tearing, or redness/yellowing of the eyes; no cough, SOB, or wheezing; no chest pain, palpitations, or edema; no abdominal pain, nausea, vomiting, reflux, melena, change in bowel movements, or rectal bleeding; no rashes, jaundice, pruritus, or skin lesions; no bruising, epistaxis, or swollen lymph nodes; no headache, dizziness, weakness, or paresthesia; no insomnia, depression, or anxiety.

Relevant History

The patient underwent an appendectomy as a child but has no other hospitalizations or medical diagnoses. He denies taking any prescription or OTC medications, herbs, vitamins, or other supplements. He had all childhood vaccines and receives annual flu shots from an urgent care clinic. His family history is significant for DM (mother and brother). The patient is married and has two young children. He is the director of sales for a local winery, working 50 hours per week, and has worked there for 17 years. He drinks 3 to 4 glasses of wine daily, which he describes as a "necessary part of my job." He has never had any work, home, or legal problems related to alcohol, and he denies binges, cravings, or withdrawal symptoms. He has never used tobacco or recreational drugs. He eats out 4 days per week: steak, potatoes, pasta, and bread. His wife cooks his favorite foods at home, including carne asada with tortillas, rice, and beans. His exercise is limited to taking his kids to a park once a week.

Allergies

None.

Medications

None.

Physical Examination

- *Vitals:* T 36.9°C (98.4°F), P 82, R 16, BP 138/84, SpO_2 99%, HT 175.26 cm (69 in.), WT 108.9 kg (240 lb), BMI 35.
- *General:* Well-developed, overnourished Latinx male, A&O×3, all vital signs stable. In no acute distress.
- *Psychiatric:* Pleasant affect, euthymic mood, fluent speech, good insight.

- *Skin, Hair, and Nails:* Skin warm and dry. Moderate palmar erythema present bilaterally. Two small spider angiomas of anterior chest but no jaundice, rashes, or varicosities noted. No abnormal findings with hair and nail exam.
- *Eyes:* PERRLA, conjunctivae clear, no scleral icterus.
- *ENT/Mouth:* No oropharyngeal lesions.
- *Neck:* Supple with no lymphadenopathy or thyromegaly.
- *Chest:* No gynecomastia or axillary lymphadenopathy noted.
- *Heart:* RRR with no murmurs, gallops, or rubs. Carotid and radial pulses are 2+ bilaterally.
- *Lungs:* Lungs CTA with no adventitious sounds noted.
- *Abdomen:* Protuberant with central adiposity and well-healed surgical scar at RLQ; no caput medusae, bulging flanks, or fluid wave present. NABS noted in all quadrants with no bruits or friction rubs. Normal areas of tympany and dullness to percussion noted. Soft, nontender; no masses or hernia appreciated. Hepatomegaly with liver span percussing to 20 cm at the mid clavicular line; palpated liver edge is firm but smooth and nontender. Spleen tip is palpable but nontender.
- *Musculoskeletal:* No muscle atrophy; trace pitting edema of BL pretibial areas; no presacral edema, clubbing, or cyanosis.
- *Neurologic:* Normal gait; no tremors or asterixis present; no focal deficits noted.
- *Diagnostic Tests:* Labs brought in by patient dated 1 month prior to visit:
  - *WBC:* 8.9×10^3/uL
  - *Hgb:* 15.0 g/dL
  - *Hct:* 44.1%
  - *MCV:* 99 fL (H)
  - *PLT:* 112×10^3/uL (L)
  - *Peripheral smear:* PLT numbers low; no clumping or giant forms; normal lymphocyte morphology
  - *BUN:* 16 mg/dL
  - *Creatinine:* 1.00 mg/dL
  - *Sodium:* 136 mmol/L
  - *Chloride:* 102 mmol/L
  - *Potassium:* 4.8 mmol/L
  - *Calcium:* 9.9 mg/dL
  - *Glucose:* 100 mg/dL (H)
  - *Albumin:* 3.6 g/dL (L)
  - *Protein:* 6.2 g/dL
  - *ALT:* 28 IU/L
  - *AST:* 40 IU/L
  - *ALP:* 141 IU/L
  - *Tbili:* 1.2 mg/dL
  - *Dbili:* 0.8 mg/dL (H)
  - *HgbA1C:* 6.0 (H)
  - *HCVAb:* negative
  - *HBsAb:* positive
  - *HBcAb:* negative
  - *HBsAg:* negative
  - *HIV Ab:* negative
  - *Total cholesterol:* 212 mg/dL (H)
  - *HDL:* 39 mg/dL (L)
  - *LDL:* 142 mg/dL (H)
  - *Trigs:* 386 mg/dL (H)

CLINICAL DISCUSSION QUESTIONS

1. What is the differential diagnosis?

2. What is the most likely diagnosis? Why?

3. Demonstrate your understanding about the pathophysiology of the most likely diagnosis.

4. Should tests/imaging studies be ordered? Which ones? Why? Think about tests/imaging beyond the primary care setting as well.

5. What are the next appropriate steps in management?

6. Demonstrate your understanding of the prevalence, screening for early intervention, and prognosis associated with the condition. Provide references to your response.

7. What are the pertinent ICD-10 and CPT (E/M) codes for this visit? Provide a short rationale.

8. What is the appropriate patient education topic for this case?

9. If not managed appropriately, what is/are the medical/legal concern(s) that may arise?

10. Think about interprofessional collaboration for this case. Provide a list of specialties or other disciplines and indicate what contribution these professionals might make to managing the patient.

BEDSIDE MANNER QUESTIONS

11. What would your communication style/approach be with this patient?

12. If the patient is distressed by the diagnosis, what might offer support?

Answers available at courseconnect.springerpub.com.

CASE 33

SKIN LESIONS AFTER SUN EXPOSURE, ADULT FEMALE

Chief Complaint

"Skin lesions after sun exposure."

History of Present Illness

A 39-year-old woman presents to her PCP for an evaluation of a rash and lesions on her face and neck that she states become worse with sun exposure. These lesions began about 12 weeks ago. She recently saw a dermatologist, who suggested she may have lupus and needed further workup for definitive diagnosis. She has returned to her PCP for a second opinion. The patient reports these lesions are itchy and, at times, painful, and they seem to heal in a few days. She also complains of moderate fatigue in the past 6 weeks but is otherwise a healthy female.

Review of Systems

The patient's ROS is positive for photosensitivity, rash on the face and neck for 12 weeks, and fatigue for 6 weeks. Her ROS is negative for headache, nausea, dyspepsia, weight loss, unexplained fever, adenopathy, oral ulcers, arthralgia, myalgia, edema, or anxiety. She denies moles of changing color.

Relevant History

The patient has a history of obesity, prediabetes, and HTN. She is up to date on vaccines, Pap smears, and dental visits.

Allergies

No known drug allergies; no known food allergies.

Medications

Hydrochlorothiazide/lisinopril 12.5 mg/10 mg QD.

Physical Examination

- *Vitals:* T 36.6°C (97.8°F), P 82, R 18, BP 143/84, HT 167.6 cm (66 in.), WT 95.7 kg (211 lb), BMI 34.1.
- *General:* No acute distress.
- *Psychiatric:* Mildly anxious.
- *Skin, Hair, and Nails:* Multiple erythematous patches and plaques with scaling noted on the face and both hands. No abnormal findings with hair or nails.
- *ENT/Mouth:* TMs clear, no lesion or ulcers noted inside the oropharyngeal mucosa.
- *Neck:* Supple, no lymphadenopathy noted.
- *Lungs:* CTA bilaterally with symmetrical chest expansion.
- *Heart:* RRR, no murmur or gallops heard.
- *Musculoskeletal:* ROM within normal limit both BL upper and lower extremity.
- *Neurologic:* A&O×3, no focal deficits noted on exam.

CLINICAL DISCUSSION QUESTIONS

1. What is the differential diagnosis?

2. What is the most likely diagnosis? Why?

3. Demonstrate your understanding about the pathophysiology of the most likely diagnosis.

4. Should tests/imaging studies be ordered? Which ones? Why? Think about tests/imaging beyond the primary care setting as well.

5. What are the next appropriate steps in management?

6. What are the risk factors and treatment options for this diagnosis? Provide references for your responses.

7. What are the pertinent ICD-10 and CPT (E/M) codes for this visit? Provide a short rationale.

8. What is the appropriate patient education topic for this case?

9. If not managed appropriately, what is/are the medical/legal concern(s) that may arise?

10. Think about interprofessional collaboration for this case. Provide a list of specialties or other disciplines and indicate what contribution these professionals might make to managing the patient.

BEDSIDE MANNER QUESTION

11. What would your communication style/approach be with this patient?

____

____

____

____

Answers available at courseconnect.springerpub.com.

NERVOUSNESS AND ANXIETY, ADULT MALE

CASE 34

Chief Complaint

"Nervousness and anxiety."

History of Present Illness

A 30-year-old man requests a same-day appointment with his PCP due to complaints of nervousness and anxiety, coupled with a profound concern that something serious was occurring related to his health. Over the past month, he has experienced excessive sweating throughout the day and at night. He also complains of mild chest discomfort, SOB, and heart palpitations. He denies pressure or heaviness in the chest, and the discomfort does not spread to his left arm, jaw, or back. There is no apparent link to physical activity. He notes that these sensations seemed similar to those his mother has reported having during a panic attack. These symptoms are new to him and have been progressively worsening over the last 2 weeks. The episodes are intermittent but come on suddenly and have left him feeling overwhelmed. Two weeks ago, he became a father to a newborn. He initially attributed his symptoms to the stress of adapting to parenthood and has noticed that his symptoms have worsened over the past 2 weeks. Despite these symptoms, he expresses contentment at home and reports doing well in his work.

Review of Systems

ROS reveals positive findings for decreased appetite, along with feelings of nausea and constipation, resulting in a weight loss of 10 lb within the last month. His ROS is negative for fever, cough, ankle swelling, flu-like symptoms, pollakiuria, polydipsia, blurry vision, blood loss, and neurologic symptoms, except for an episodic headache which he rates as 6/10 in intensity. He denies any thoughts of suicide, delirium, or psychotic symptoms.

Relevant History

The patient typically enjoys good health with no significant past medical history. His family medical history does include systemic HTN and T2DM in his father. His mother has a history of panic attacks. There is no reported family history of cancer or endocrinology diseases. Regarding lifestyle habits, he is a nonsmoker, drinks two cups of coffee in the morning, and consumes four to six beers only during the weekends. He does not use illicit drugs or take any muscle-building supplements. He leads an active lifestyle—often participating in activities such as playing hockey with friends, going to the gym, biking, and skiing. His diet is healthy, and he generally has a good appetite. He has been living with his wife for 2 years and became a father to a newborn weeks ago, which he is happy about. He finds fulfillment in his job within the bank industry and reports no significant stress at work.

Allergies

No known drug allergies; no known food allergies.

Medications

Occasional OTC medications (e.g., acetaminophen).

PHYSICAL EXAMINATION

- *Vitals:* T: 37.4°C (99.3°F), P 98 (regular), RR 22, SpO_2 100%
- *BP measurements:* Right arm 200/105 mmHg and 190/100 mmHg after 10 minutes of rest. Left arm 198/105 mm Hg and 196/103 mmHg after 10 minutes of rest.
- *Anthropometric measurement:* WT 85 kg (187.39 lb; last year his WT was 197 lb), HT 190 cm (74.8 in.), BMI 23.5.
- *General:* The patient appears pale, nervous, agitated, short of breath while speaking, speaks faster than usual, and exhibits a light tremor in both hands.
- *Skin, Hair, and Nails:* Skin pallor, excessive sweating on his back, and no peripheral edema.
- *Eyes:* Normal vision and no exophthalmos.
- *ENT/Mouth:* Normal, no cyanosis
- *Neck:* Normal ROM, no palpable masses in the thyroid region.
- *Lungs:* CTA BL: no rales, crackles, or wheezing detected.
- *Heart:* Regular rapid HR. CTA, no abnormal beats or murmurs.
- *Abdomen:* Soft, tender to palpation in the upper abdomen and slight discomfort upon renal palpation on both sides. No palpable abdominal mass.
- *Neurologic:* Normal, aside from light tremors in both arms.

Psychiatric Exam

- *Mood and affect:* Anxious
- *Speech:* Clear, coherent, slightly increased speed rate and volume
- *Thought content:* Reports symptoms of anxiety (emotional concerns regarding health and physical symptoms including feelings of restlessness). He reports an absence of depressive symptoms, delusions, hallucinations, or paranoid beliefs and has no signs of mania. No presence of suicidal or homicidal ideations. Insight and judgment are within normal limits.

CLINICAL DISCUSSION QUESTIONS

1. What is the differential diagnosis?

2. What is the most likely diagnosis? Why?

3. Demonstrate your understanding about the pathophysiology of the most likely diagnosis.

4. Should tests/imaging studies be ordered? Which ones? Why? Think about tests/imaging beyond the primary care setting as well.

5. What are the next appropriate steps in management?

6. What are the treatment options for this diagnosis? Provide references for your response.

7. What are the pertinent ICD-10 and CPT (E/M) codes for this visit? Provide a short rationale.

8. What is the appropriate patient education topic for this case?

9. If not managed appropriately, what is/are the medical/legal concern(s) that may arise?

10. Think about interprofessional collaboration for this case. Provide a list of specialties or other disciplines and indicate what contribution these professionals might make to managing the patient.

BEDSIDE MANNER QUESTION

11. What would your communication style/approach be with this patient?

Answers available at courseconnect.springerpub.com.

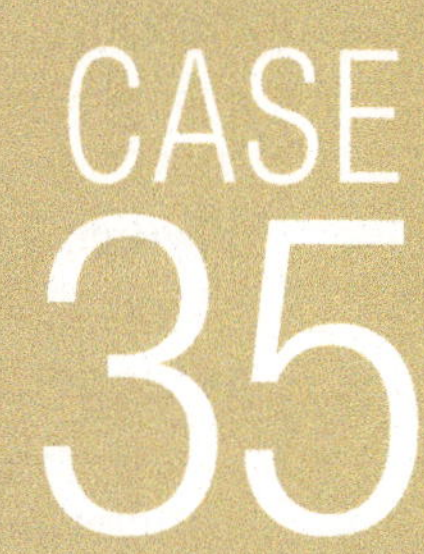

FATIGUE AND JOINT ACHES, ADULT MALE

Chief Complaint

"Fatigue and joint aches."

History of Present Illness

A 55-year-old man presents to a free clinic complaining of fatigue, headache, and muscle and joint aches. The patient states he was seen at the clinic 1 month ago with the same symptoms and was diagnosed with a viral infection and instructed in supportive care, including oral hydration and acetaminophen. The symptoms began 2 to 3 months ago. He thinks he has a fever but has not checked the temperature. Aspirin has not helped. His muscle and joint aches are diffuse. There is no joint swelling or erythema. His headache is in the temple and occipital region, the pain is constant, and the patient denies photo-or phonophobia. He denies any recent injuries and has no sick contacts.

Review of Systems

The ROS is positive for a 15-lb weight loss over the past 2 months and swollen lymph nodes in his groin and armpits. The ROS was negative for chills, sweats, nausea and vomiting, rash, SOB, chest pain, abdominal pain, or weakness.

Relevant History

The patient's medical history is positive for HTN that is presently untreated. He has no surgical history. His social history includes consuming an occasional beer, but he denies smoking or IV drug abuse. The patient worked as an accountant but lost his job 5 years ago. He lives in a homeless shelter and works as a janitor. His family history is positive for mother dying at age 65 due to renal failure as a complication of DM; his father died at age 72 from an MI. His brothers are alive and well at ages 60 and 58.

Allergies

No known drug allergies; no known food allergies.

Medications

Acetaminophen 500 mg every 6 hours PRN for fever.

Physical Examination

- *Vitals:* T 38.1°C (100.6°F), P 102, R 20, BP 149/89, WT 61.7 kg (136 lb), HT 177.8 cm (70 in.), BMI 19.5.
- *General:* A 55-year-old man who appears older than his stated age; he appears tired, thin, and without energy.
- *Psychiatric:* Appears tired but no signs of depression or anxiety.
- *Skin, Hair, and Nails:* Skin is warm and dry; fingernails are smooth and shiny, transparent, and normally curved. Hair distribution shows male pattern baldness; remaining hair is thick with normal luster.
- *Eyes:* Corneas are clear. Conjunctivas are moist and without discharge; small red spots are seen on the conjunctiva. Disc margins are sharp, arterioles are bright red with a narrow light reflex, and there is no tapering or nicking noted. There are no hemorrhages or exudates.

- *ENT/Mouth:* Auricles are nontender. Canals are patent; the TMs are intact; no bulging or erythema noted.
- *Neck:* There is no swelling or tenderness noted in the pre- or post auricular nodes and posterior cervical, anterior cervical, or supraclavicular nodes.
- *Lungs:* Breath sounds are heard throughout the lungs, symmetric, and vesicular. Breath sounds are low pitched and of soft intensity. No adventitious sounds are noted.
- *Heart:* RRR. There is a grade IV/VI holosystolic murmur in the mitral region that radiates to the left axilla; a loud S3 and audible S4.
- *Abdomen:* On inspection, the abdomen is symmetric; skin is smooth and soft without striae. No bulges, peristalsis, or pulsations are visible. On auscultation, clicks and gurgles are heard 10 to 15 times per minute; no hums, bruits, or friction rubs are heard. On percussions, the liver size is 6 cm midsternal line and 9 cm midclavicular line. There is no tenderness on light or deep palpation. The spleen tip can be palpated 2 cm below the costal margin on deep inspiration. There is no tenderness to light or deep palpation. No referred pain or rebound tenderness.
- *Lymphatic:* There are several tender lymph nodes in the axilla bilaterally and there are moderate-sized, tender inguinal lymph nodes bilaterally.
- *Musculoskeletal:* There are no areas of heat, tenderness, or soft tissue thickening; no fluid in the joints. Some tenderness is noted with movement of the knees.
- *Neurologic:* A&O×3; cranial nerves II to XII are grossly intact.

Clinical Discussion Questions

1. What is the differential diagnosis?

____

____

____

____

2. What is the most likely diagnosis? Why?

____

____

____

____

3. Demonstrate your understanding about the pathophysiology of the most likely diagnosis.

____

____

____

____

4. Should tests/imaging studies be ordered? Which ones? Why? Think about tests/imaging beyond the primary care setting as well.

5. What are the next appropriate steps in management?

6. What are the causes, risk factors, diagnosis, and treatments of the diagnosis? Provide references for your response.

7. What are the pertinent ICD-10 and CPT (E/M) codes for this visit? Provide a short rationale.

8. What is the appropriate patient education topic for this case?

9. If not managed appropriately, what is/are the medical/legal concern(s) that may arise?

10. Think about interprofessional collaboration for this case. Provide a list of specialties or other disciplines and indicate what contribution these professionals might make to managing the patient.

BEDSIDE MANNER QUESTION

11. What would your communication style/approach be with this patient?

Answers available at courseconnect.springerpub.com.

CASE 36

UNEXPLAINED WEIGHT LOSS, ADULT FEMALE

Chief Complaint

"Unexplained weight loss."

History of Present Illness

A 36-year-old woman presents to her PCP with multiple complaints: weight loss and palpitations worsened by anxiety about her health for the last 3 months. She states she has been the sole caretaker for her ill mother for the last 6 months and had no time for herself or time to seek care. She states she was noticing a weight loss of 15 lb (6.8 kg) continuing even though she has been indulging in nervous eating habits, especially when she is stressed. The patient states she is stressed and anxious about her health after witnessing how Alzheimer disease is affecting her mother. The patient attributes her palpitations to anxiety about her health and her mother's health.

Review of Systems

The ROS was positive for weight loss, palpitations, and anxiety and negative for sweating, heat intolerance, tremors, headache, change of vision, chest pain, SOB, fever, chills, vomiting, diarrhea, constipation, or suicidal ideation.

Relevant History

The patient's history is significant for a negative screening of depression and anxiety done last year during a physical exam. She is not a smoker. She has a 12-pack-year smoking history but had quit 5 years ago. There is no substance abuse history (neither alcohol or drugs). She is sexually active and in a monogamous relationship with her husband of 10 years. She reports she is happy with her husband and children. Her family history is positive for DM, HTN, and CAD.

Allergies

No known drug allergies; no known food allergies.

Medications

Melatonin 4 mg PRN for sleep.

Physical Examination

- *Vitals:* T 37.2°C (98.9°F), P 102, R 18, BP 130/78, WT 101.6 kg (224 lb), HT 170 cm (67 in.), BMI 35.
- *General:* Appears anxious and fatigued; mild acute distress.
- *Psychiatric:* Mildly anxious, scored negative on PHQ-9 and GAD-7.
- *Eyes:* Mild exophthalmos with PERRL, EOMI. BL conjunctival inflammation noted.
- *Neck:* Soft, nontender, slightly and diffusely enlarged thyroid without lymphadenopathy.
- *Heart:* Tachycardic, S1 and S2 present without murmur or gallop.
- *Lungs:* CTA bilaterally, good air movement throughout.
- *Abdomen:* Soft, nondistended, and moderately tender throughout.
- *Extremities:* No BL swelling.
- *Neurologic:* A&O×3, CN II to XII intact.

CLINICAL DISCUSSION QUESTIONS

1. What is the differential diagnosis?

2. What is the most likely diagnosis? Why?

3. Demonstrate your understanding about the pathophysiology of the most likely diagnosis.

4. Should tests/imaging studies be ordered? Which ones? Why? Think about tests/imaging beyond the primary care setting as well.

5. What are the next appropriate steps in management?

6. What are the cause and clinical manifestations of the diagnosis? Provide references for your response.

7. What are the pertinent ICD-10 and CPT (E/M) codes for this visit? Provide a short rationale.

8. What is the appropriate patient education topic for this case?

9. If not managed appropriately, what is/are the medical/legal concern(s) that may arise?

10. Think about interprofessional collaboration for this case. Provide a list of specialties or other disciplines and indicate what contribution these professionals might make to managing the patient.

BEDSIDE MANNER QUESTIONS

11. What would your communication style/approach be with this patient?

12. If a patient is distressed by the diagnosis, what might offer support?

____

____

____

____

Answers available at courseconnect.springerpub.com.

CASE 37

PAINFUL LUMP IN ARMPIT, ADULT FEMALE

Chief Complaint

"Painful lump in armpit."

History of Present Illness

A 23-year-old woman with no significant medical history is brought to her PCP by her boyfriend who is worried about "a really painful lump in her armpit that is not going away." The patient states she noticed a small, rubbery bump that appeared in the center of her left axilla approximately 4 days ago. She thought a pimple was developing as she reports developing them occasionally after shaving with her boyfriend's razor. This one pimple, she states, is getting larger, seems to be spreading, and is very painful.

She reports slight chills and a fever that started this morning but has not taken her temperature. She admits to a stinging, burning, 9/10 pain in her left axilla, extending into her left inner elbow with any movement of her left UE. She denies numbness or tingling of her left hand and fingers. Being right-hand dominant, she reports trying not to use her left arm as the pain intensifies with movement, especially noticed when trying to apply deodorant today. She has tried OTC ibuprofen which she states has helped little to reduce the pain that is interfering with her sleep. Her last dose of two 200 mg tablets was at 11 p.m. last night. She does not recall when her last tetanus immunization was, neither can she recall that this issue has ever been this worrisome before. She denies exposure to new perfumes, colognes, soaps, detergents, or dyes.

Review of Systems

The patient's ROS is positive for subjective fever, chills, fatigue, and insomnia for 1 day due to painful left axilla. ROS is also positive for painful, erythematous mass in her left axilla for 4 days; pain extends to elbow, sparing left hand and fingers. Her ROS is negative for unintentional weight loss, weakness, numbness, tingling, or paralysis of the left UE.

Relevant History

The patient had acute appendicitis with a resultant laparoscopic appendectomy at age 17. Her last menstrual period was 2 months ago—she experiences menses four times per year secondary to birth control taken. She is a social smoker (5 to 6 cigarettes on weekends) and has 1 to 2 vodka/energy drinks per weekend. She denies recreational or illicit drug use. Her family history is noncontributory.

Allergies

No known drug allergies; no known food allergies.

Medications

- Extended-cycle birth control pills, one tablet QD.
- Ibuprofen, two 200 mg tablets PO PRN for left axillary pain.

Physical Examination

- *Vitals:* T 37.7°C (99.8°F), P 88, R 14, BP 128/72, HT 170.2 cm (67 in.), WT 62 kg (136 lb), BMI 21.3.

- *General:* A well-nourished young adult female of stated age is found sitting on the examination table in slight discomfort. She is A&O×3.
- *Skin, Hair, and Nails:* Deeply seated, cord-like nodular and elongated 4 cm × 1 cm left axillary mass that is erythematous, tender, and swollen, extending distally to the left anterior breast. Mass is slightly fluctuant at its center with multiple pointing white heads, diffusely warm. The skin surrounding the mass is slightly hard to palpation. No lacerations, open lesions, or drainage. No skin lesions or lacerations on any other area of the patient's body.
- *Neck:* FROM, cervical and tonsillar lymphadenopathy, L > R.
- *Breasts:* Firm, slightly pendulous, symmetric bilaterally, without nipple discharge or retraction. Tender left tail of Spence, extending proximally to erythematous left axillary mass.
- *Lungs:* CTA bilaterally, without wheezes.
- *Heart:* RRR without murmurs, rubs, or gallops.
- *Peripheral Vascular:* Extremities warm throughout, BUE and BLE pulses 2+ and symmetric. Capillary refill brisk, less than 2 seconds throughout. Upper and lower distal extremities without edema. No varicosities.
- *Musculoskeletal:* FROM of right UE. LROM left shoulder, eliciting severe pain with left UE extension overhead with external rotation. FROM left elbow, wrist, hand, and fingers.
- *Neurologic:* CN II to XII grossly intact. UE and LE sensation intact to light and sharp touch. Muscle bulk, tone, 5/5 strength symmetric throughout. BL brachioradialis and patellar reflexes 2+/symmetric.

CLINICAL DISCUSSION QUESTIONS

1. What is the differential diagnosis?

2. What is the most likely diagnosis? Why?

3. Demonstrate your understanding about the pathophysiology of the most likely diagnosis.

4. Should tests/imaging studies be ordered? Which ones? Why? Think about tests/imaging beyond the primary care setting as well.

5. What are the next appropriate steps in management?

6. What are the exacerbation factors, diagnosis, and treatment of the diagnosis? Provide references for your responses.

7. What are the pertinent ICD-10 and CPT (E/M) codes for this visit? Provide a short rationale.

8. What is the appropriate patient education topic for this case?

9. If not managed appropriately, what is/are the medical/legal concern(s) that may arise?

10. Think about interprofessional collaboration for this case. Provide a list of specialties or other disciplines and indicate what contribution these professionals might make to managing the patient.

Bedside Manner Question

11. What would your communication style/approach be with this patient?

Answers available at courseconnect.springerpub.com.

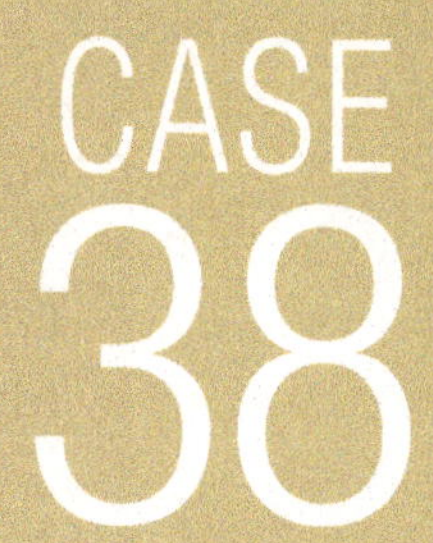

DIABETES CHECK, ADULT MALE

Chief Complaint

"Diabetes check."

History of Present Illness

A 58-year-old Latinx man presents to a new PCP to check on his DM status. His last annual visit was almost 3 years ago and it has been 6 months since his last DM visit. The patient states that he used to see a "specialist for his kidney" but stopped going and wants to initiate care here due to his insurance. He was diagnosed with DM almost 5 years ago (cannot recall exact year), and he has been taking metformin 500 mg BID for his DM most days (some days he forgets to take it). He has been taking atorvastatin 40 mg QD for his high cholesterol. He was also previously told he has high BP. He was started on a medication for his BP but stopped taking because he felt OK without it. The patient admits he does not keep appointments well and he used to be on insulin prior; however, he was not adherent. He states cost as the barrier that kept him from adhering to his medication regimen. He now has active insurance. His diet consists of red meats, fast food, rice, beans, and potatoes. He also complains of chronic fatigue and headaches that are intermittent but occur more frequently now and are worse in severity. The headache is located in the occipital region and radiates to the temporal regions. The patient describes the pain as a throbbing and pulsating sensation. He notes some eye blurriness and nausea at times and thinks he drinks more than what he voids but has no difficulty voiding.

Review of Systems

The patient's ROS is positive for fatigue, nausea, urine retention, and occipital headache. Pertinent negatives are aura, vomiting, sudden vision changes or loss, or halos. He denies cognitive problems, angina, SOB, diaphoresis, palpitations, or extremity swelling. He further denies polydipsia, polyphagia, polyuria, dysuria, hematuria, discharge, hesitancy, frequency, or dribbling.

Relevant History

The patient's history is significant for HTN, T2DM, and hyperlipidemia. He has a family history of HTN, DM (type unknown), and hyperlipidemia. He is a field worker, is married, and has two children.

Allergies

No known drug allergies; no known food allergies.

Medications

- Metformin 500 mg BID.
- Atorvastatin 40 mg QD.

Physical Examination

- *Vitals:* T 36.8°C (98.2°F), P 92, R 16, BP 178/106, HT 170.18 cm (67 in.),WT 83 kg (183 lb), BMI 28.66.
- *General:* Alert, well hydrated, in no distress, well developed, well nourished.
- *Psychiatric:* Cognitive function intact, cooperative with exam, good eye contact.
- *Eyes:* EOMI, PERRLA.

- *Neck:* Supple, FROM, no cervical lymphadenopathy, no thyromegaly.
- *Chest:* Normal shape and expansion.
- *Lungs:* CTA bilaterally, good air movement.
- *Heart:* RRR, no jugular vein distention or murmurs.
- *Abdomen:* Active BS ×4, no distention, nontender with no rebound, soft on palpation.
- *Musculoskeletal:* Mild pitting edema bilaterally 1+, pedal pulses 2+ bilaterally, no clubbing, cyanosis.
- *Neurologic:* Nonfocal, A&O×3, normal gait. CN II to XII grossly intact.

Clinical Discussion Questions

1. What is the differential diagnosis?

2. What is the most likely diagnosis? Why?

3. Demonstrate your understanding about the pathophysiology of the most likely diagnosis.

4. Should tests/imaging studies be ordered? Which ones? Why? Think about tests/imaging beyond the primary care setting as well.

5. What are the next appropriate steps in management?

6. Using credible literature, explain whether Latinx patients are at a greater or lesser risk for this diagnosis and why. Provide references for your responses.

7. What are the pertinent ICD-10 and CPT (E/M) codes for this visit? Provide a short rationale.

8. What is the appropriate patient education topic for this case?

9. If not managed appropriately, what is/are the medical/legal concern(s) that may arise?

10. Think about interprofessional collaboration for this case. Provide a list of specialties or other disciplines and indicate what contribution these professionals might make to managing the patient.

BEDSIDE MANNER QUESTIONS

11. What would your communication style/approach be with this patient?

12. If a patient is distressed by the diagnosis, what might offer support?

Answers available at courseconnect.springerpub.com.

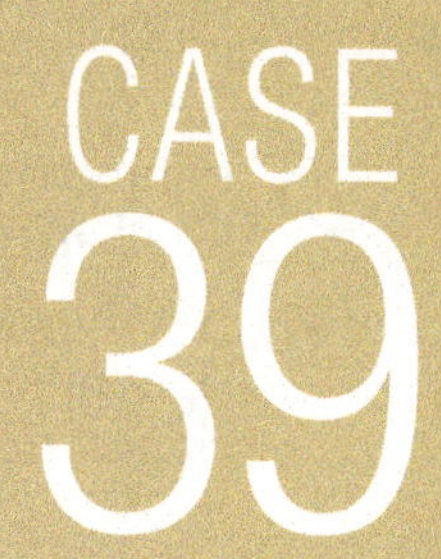

BILATERAL HEEL PAIN, ADULT FEMALE

Chief Complaint

"Bilateral heel pain."

History of Present Illness

A 28-year-old woman with obesity presents as a new patient with a several-month history of BL heel pain. She denies any precipitating event, trauma, or specific incident that triggered her pain. The patient describes the heel pain as a sharp and stabbing sensation, exacerbated by prolonged standing and walking. The patient reports that the heel pain begins after taking the first few steps after getting out of bed.

A local urgent care provider diagnosed the patient with overuse syndrome and prescribed ibuprofen, rest, and OTC inserts for her shoes. However, the patient reported minimal relief in her symptoms. She works as a grocery clerk and is on her feet 8 hours a day.

Review of Systems

The patient's ROS is positive for heel pain with prolonged standing and walking. Additionally, she experiences pain at night. The patient's ROS is negative for bilateral swelling of the ankle, foot, and digits. She denies any altered sensation or weakness in both extremities. She also denies any gait abnormalities or flat feet, any temperature changes, any recent illnesses, or hospitalizations.

Relevant History

The patient's medical history is unremarkable other than obesity. She works in a local grocery as a grocery clerk. She is single and currently not sexually active. She does not drink alcohol or use any recreational drugs. Her family history is noncontributory.

Medications

Ibuprofen 200 mg 1 or 2 tablets Q6h PRN for pain.

Allergies

No known drug allergies; no known food allergies.

Physical Examination

- *Vitals:* T 37°C (98.6°F), P 84, R 20, BP 134/88, HT 167.6 cm (66 in.), WT 112.5 kg. (248 lb), BMI 40.
- *General:* No apparent distress.
- *Musculoskeletal/Bilateral Foot and Ankle:* There is no swelling, deformity, crepitus, or bogginess of the feet and ankle. There are no skin changes. There is no tenderness over the forefoot and midfoot foot. ROM is as follows: dorsiflexion 15/15, plantar flexion 40/40, eversion 20/20, inversion 35/35, all without pain or discomfort. An anterior drawer test is negative. There is no lateral ligamentous laxity. There is mild hallux valgus deformity to both the great toes without tenderness. There is a negative Tinel sign over the tibial and sural nerves. There is moderate pes cavus of both feet. There is no forefoot varus or "too many toes sign." There is no hindfoot valgus. There is no tenderness over the subtalar joint. There is exquisite point tenderness over the medial aspect of the calcaneal tuberosity. Heels are

symmetrical without any bony masses palpated. Dorsalis pedis and posterior tibialis are 2+. Capillary refill is less than 2 seconds.

- *Neurologic:* Sensation intact to the dorsal and plantar aspects of the foot, ankle, and leg. No signs of foot drop. No altered sensation compared to the contralateral extremity. No ankle clonus. Achilles reflex 2+.

Clinical Discussion Questions

1. What is the differential diagnosis?

2. What is the most likely diagnosis? Why?

3. Demonstrate your understanding of the pathophysiology of the most likely diagnosis.

4. Should tests/imaging studies be ordered? Which ones? Why? Think about tests/imaging beyond the primary care setting as well.

5. What are the next appropriate steps in management?

6. Review a reliable, recent reference and demonstrate an understanding of the treatment recommendations associated with this diagnosis. Include the name of the references.

7. What are the pertinent ICD-10 and CPT (E/M) codes for this visit? Provide a short rationale.

8. What is the appropriate patient education topic for this case?

9. If not managed appropriately, what is/are the medical/legal concern(s) that may arise?

10. Think about interprofessional collaboration for this case. Provide a list of specialties or other disciplines and indicate what contribution these professionals might make to managing the patient.

BEDSIDE MANNER QUESTION

11. What would your communication style/approach be with this patient?

Answers available at courseconnect.springerpub.com.

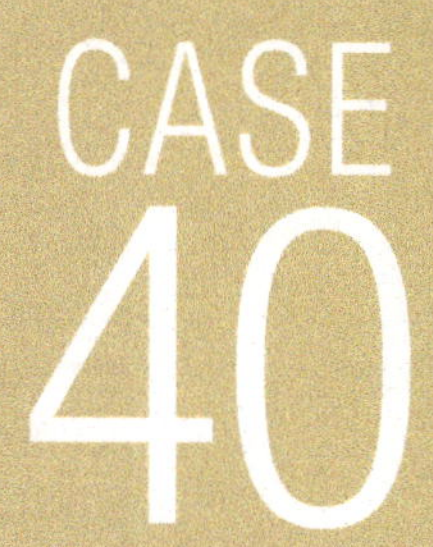

EYE INJURY, ADULT MALE

Chief Complaint

"Eye injury."

History of Present Illness

A 32-year-old man presents to the clinic complaining of getting something in his OS that he feels is still there. Just prior to presenting, he was stretching a bungee cord across the top of his kayak to secure it to the roof racks of his car, when the bungee cord snapped in half, ricocheting the rubber cord with the metal S hook toward his face. He reports something hitting his OS as he could not get out of the way fast enough, has tried looking in a mirror to see if he could see what was in his eye, and has tried to flush out whatever might be stuck in his eye using all 16 oz of his bottled water. He reports the OS pain as 10/10, stinging, sharp, throbbing, and very sensitive to light. He complains also of very blurry vision in the OS, not being able to make much out, including shapes. He denies double vision, any eye injury in the past, or the use of wear corrective lenses of any kind. He has not had eye surgery and cannot recall his last tetanus immunization. He has not taken anything to alleviate the pain other than to hold an ice pack over his OS. He denies any other injury to his face, mouth, or teeth. He is here with his wife.

Review of Systems

The patient's ROS is positive for foreign body sensation in the OS with severe pain, photosensitivity, excessive tearing, redness and extreme blurred vision OS, and throbbing headache behind OS. His ROS is negative for double vision, spots, specks, flashing lights, corrective lenses, facial lacerations, abrasions, or head injury.

Relevant History

The patient has no contributory medical or surgical history. He is happily married and the father of two children. He is a social drinker. He denies tobacco or drug use. His family history is noncontributory.

Allergies

Sulfonamides create rash and intense pruritis; no known food allergies.

Medications

Multivitamin PO QD.

Physical Examination

- *Vitals:* T 37.2°C (99.0°F), P 114, R 16, BP 148/94, HT 185.4 cm (73 in.), WT 86.2 kg (190 lb), BMI 25.1.
- *General:* Frightened male of stated age, worried about OS vision. A&O; answers all questions appropriately.
- *Skin, Hair, and Nails:* Warm throughout; no lesions, lacerations, ecchymosis. No abnormal findings with hair or nails.
- *Head:* Atraumatic, normocephalic, nontender.

- *Eyes:* No periorbital lacerations, lesions, ecchymosis, step offs, or tenderness bilaterally.
  - *OS:* Swollen and tender upper and lower lids, good position, unable to close fully. Injected sclera and hyperemic conjunctiva, subconjunctival hemorrhage at the medial canthus extending to the iris, excessive tearing, teardrop-shaped pupil not reactive to light or accommodation. Foreign body not visible to the naked eye. No fluid visualized as being emitted from the anterior or lateral portions of the globe. EOMs limited in movement. Difficult to assess retinal structures funduscopically due to patient's pain level and difficulty with visualization.
  - *OD:* No lid edema, good position and closure, injected sclera, pink conjunctive. Pupil 4 mm, round, reactive to light and accommodation. EOMIs intact, no disc edema or swelling, venous pulsations, or AV nicking.
- *ENT/Mouth:* Hearing acuity intact bilaterally to whispered voice. No deformities, lacerations, lesions, or tenderness externally, bilaterally. TMs pearly gray, positive cone of light; no discharge or bleeding bilaterally. No maxillary or frontal sinus tenderness. Nares patent, septum midline, dark pink mucosa with clear nasal drainage L>R. Teeth and gums in good repair; no bleeding. Oral mucosa and tongue without lesions or lacerations, oropharynx patent, tonsils 1+ and symmetric, uvula midline.
- *Neck:* FROM, supple, no adenopathy.
- *Neurologic:* CN II grossly intact OD; unable to assess CN II OS due to extreme blurred vision. CN III to XII grossly intact.

CLINICAL DISCUSSION QUESTIONS

1. What is the differential diagnosis?

2. What is the most likely diagnosis? Why?

3. Demonstrate your understanding about the pathophysiology of the most likely diagnosis.

4. Should tests/imaging studies be ordered? Which ones? Why? Think about tests/imaging beyond the primary care setting as well.

5. What are the next appropriate steps in management?

6. What are the treatment approaches, prevalence, and physical exam techniques of this diagnosis? Provide references for your responses.

7. What are the pertinent ICD-10 and CPT (E/M) codes for this visit? Provide a short rationale.

8. What is the appropriate patient education topic for this case?

9. If not managed appropriately, what is/are the medical/legal concern(s) that may arise?

10. Think about interprofessional collaboration for this case. Provide a list of specialties or other disciplines and indicate what contribution these professionals might make to managing the patient.

BEDSIDE MANNER QUESTIONS

11. What would your communication style/approach be with this patient and his wife?

12. If a patient and his wife are distressed by the diagnosis, what might offer support?

Answers available at courseconnect.springerpub.com.

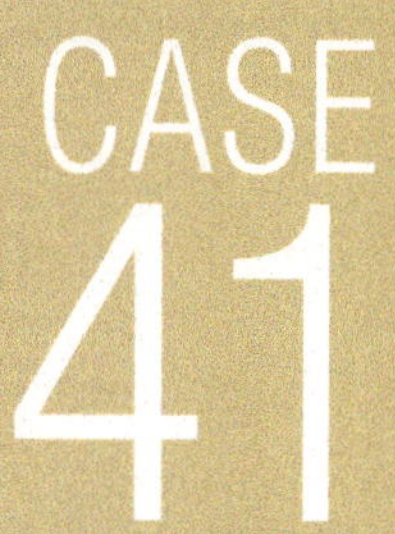

LUMP IN THROAT, ADULT MALE

Chief Complaint

"Lump in throat."

History of Present Illness

A 35-year-old man arrives at his PCP's office reporting the sensation of a lump in his throat for over 1 month and episodes of mild epigastric pain with occasional nausea. He has experienced bloating and belching. He has a dry cough and feels like he needs to clear his throat often. He has a sour taste in his mouth and states that he frequently gets painful canker sores. He also complains of a burning type of pain to the anterior chest. The burning pain starts in the upper chest area and works its way up to the neck and throat area. He experiences the symptoms daily, and they become worse when he lies down or after eating.

Review of Systems

The patient's ROS is positive for nausea, bloating, belching, cough, canker sores, chest pain, and repetitive throat clearing. His ROS is negative for sore throat, hoarseness, dysphagia, vomiting, abdominal pain, melena, weight loss, change in appetite, asthma, ear pain, tooth pain, or exertional type chest pain. He denies a cardiac history or HTN. He does not smoke. He occasionally drinks alcohol and daily drinks caffeinated soda. He denies any SOB or wheezing.

Relevant History

The patient has a history of Paget Schroetter syndrome at age 25. He is a full-time high school teacher. He exercises regularly. He is sexually active in a long-term relationship with his live-in girlfriend. His family history includes both grandparents with DM and HTN. His father, who is living, has a history of stage 4 throat cancer at age 55.

Allergies

No known drug allergies; no known food allergies.

Medications

None.

Physical Examination

- *Vitals:* T 37.2°C (98.8°F), P 82, R 20, BP 120/80, HT 193 cm (76 in.), WT 127 kg (280 lb), BMI 34.08.
- *General:* Alert and cooperative. Sitting comfortably on the exam table. Well nourished. No acute distress.
- *Psychiatric:* Mildly anxious.
- *ENT/Mouth:* TMs clear; canals clear bilaterally. Nose with no nasal septal deviation; mucous membranes moist and pink. Throat with pink and moist oropharynx; no erythema, no tonsillar enlargement, no lesions, no tooth erosion. Mouth with no sores or lesions present.
- *Neck:* Supple with no lymphadenopathy; thyroid normal size.
- *Chest:* Symmetric with no palpated tenderness.

- *Lungs:* CTA bilaterally; no rales, wheezes, or rhonchi.
- *Heart:* RRR; no murmurs or gallops.
- *Abdomen:* Nondistended and soft with NABS present in all quadrants; no pain on palpation of the abdomen.

CLINICAL DISCUSSION QUESTIONS

1. What is the differential diagnosis?

2. What is the most likely diagnosis? Why?

3. Demonstrate your understanding about the pathophysiology of the most likely diagnosis.

4. Should tests/imaging studies be ordered? Which ones? Why? Think about tests/imaging beyond the primary care setting as well.

5. What are the next appropriate steps in management?

6. What is the prevalence and treatment approach of the diagnosis and the risks associated with the medications when used long term? Provide references(s) for your response.

7. What are the pertinent ICD-10 and CPT (E/M) codes for this visit? Provide a short rationale.

8. What is the appropriate patient education topic for this case?

9. If not managed appropriately, what is/are the medical/legal concern(s) that may arise?

10. Think about interprofessional collaboration for this case. Provide a list of specialties or other disciplines and indicate what contribution these professionals might make to managing the patient.

Bedside Manner Question

11. What would your communication style/approach be with this patient?

____

____

____

____

Answers available at courseconnect.springerpub.com.

CASE 42

EXTREME WEAKNESS, ADULT MALE

Chief Complaint

"Extreme weakness."

History of Present Illness

A 22-year-old Vietnamese male was carried into his PCP's office by two male family members. The family members told the nurse the patient is weak and unable to walk on his own. The patient had immigrated to the United States from Vietnam 2 years ago and has no previously diagnosed major medical problems. His weakness started yesterday, initially as muscle cramps, which gradually progressed to generalized muscle weakness. He denied any muscle pain and has had no associated symptoms. He denied any injury and any psychiatric problems. The patient mentioned that the weakness started in his LE first and then gradually progressed to his UE. He denied any breathing problems. The patient also stated that he was at a birthday party the day before his symptoms started and he ate a large meal containing rice.

Review of Systems

The patient's ROS is positive for generalized muscle weakness, fatigue, and muscle cramps; he is unable to walk. His ROS is negative for any recent weight loss, fever, chills, nausea, vomiting, headaches or URI symptoms, SOB, chest pain, or abdominal pain. The review is also negative for any urinary symptoms or mood changes or depression.

Relevant History

The patient is Vietnamese and has only been in the United States a few years. He has occasional mild seasonal asthma. He smokes half a pack of cigarettes a day. Once a week, he has one or two beers. He denies any THC or illicit drug use. He lives with his older brother in an apartment. He works as a store clerk at a convenience store and has no unusual stress at work. He has no girlfriend at this time and has not been sexually active for a few months. His father had a heart attack at age 50; his mother is healthy. Both live in Vietnam. His older brother had been hospitalized for an unknown medical condition.

Allergies

No known drug or food allergies.

Medications

None.

Physical Examination

- *Vitals:* T 98.2°F (36.8°C), BP 128/74, P 110, R 12, SPO_2 98%, WT 72.57 kg (160 lb), HT 172.7 cm (68 in.), BMI 24.3.
- *General:* Appeared anxious and weak but in no other distress. Nontoxic.
- *Psychiatric:* Normal mood and affect.
- *Skin, Hair, and Nails:* Clear with no rashes, lesions, or petechiae or purpura. No abnormal findings with hair or nails.
- *ENT/Mouth:* TM clear bilaterally, no discharge in the ears, oral mucosa moist, no pharyngeal erythema.

- *Neck:* Soft and supple with no nuchal rigidity or thyromegaly.
- *Chest:* Adequate and symmetric chest expansion.
- *Lungs:* Clear bilaterally with no wheezing, rales, or rhonchi.
- *Heart:* Mild tachycardia but regular with no murmurs or gallops.
- *Abdomen*: Soft. Nontender. No palpable masses or organomegaly. BS normal.
- *Lymphatic*: No palpable lymphadenopathy symmetrically.
- *Musculoskeletal*: Patient had diffuse muscle weakness at 2/5 of all his large muscle groups in all extremities. No muscle tenderness. He was unable to walk due to generalized weakness.
- *Neurologic:* A&O×3. CN II to XII grossly normal. No detectable sensory deficits. DTRs 1+ bilaterally; decreased symmetrically.

Clinical Discussion Questions

1. What is the differential diagnosis?

2. What is the most likely diagnosis? Why?

3. Demonstrate your understanding about the pathophysiology of most likely diagnosis.

4. Should tests/imaging studies be ordered? Which ones? Why? Think about tests/imaging beyond the primary care setting as well.

5. What are the next appropriate steps in management?

6. What are the triggers, associated conditions, and treatment approaches for the diagnosis? Provide references for your responses.

7. What are the pertinent ICD-10 and CPT (E/M) codes for this visit? Provide a short rationale.

8. What is the appropriate patient education topic for this case?

9. If not managed appropriately, what is/are the medical/legal concern(s) that may arise?

10. Think about interprofessional collaboration for this case. Provide a list of specialties or other disciplines and indicate what contribution these professionals might make to managing the patient.

BEDSIDE MANNER QUESTION

11. What would your communication style/approach be with this patient?

Answers available at courseconnect.springerpub.com.

CASE 43

PAIN AND REDNESS IN BREAST, ADULT FEMALE

Chief Complaint

"Pain and redness in the breast."

History of Present Illness

A 50-year-old Black woman presents to her PCP with a complaint of persistent pain and redness in her left breast for the past week. She reports she first noticed the pain 4 weeks ago; however, she did not notice any skin changes at the time. One week later, she started noticing redness of the skin near and around her nipple, which made her concerned about infection. She went to a local urgent care, where she was diagnosed with cellulitis of the breast and was prescribed a 7-day course of cephalexin. She has since completed the medication and has not seen any improvement, despite taking the medication as directed and to completion. She has not noticed any worsening of the pain since it started or noticed it to be spreading.

When asked about the pain and the redness, she states that it felt and looked very similar to a bout of mastitis she experienced while breastfeeding her son years ago. She rates the pain at 6/10 and describes it as intermittent and worsened by touching the breast or with any applied pressure (like wearing her bra). She has been unable to wear her bra due to the discomfort. She denies any itching of the area and describes the pain as dull, burning, and achy without radiation beyond the breast. She denies any new exposures, including no new lotions, soaps, detergents, clothing, or foods. She denies any similar symptoms in or on her right breast. She admits to routinely performing self-breast exams at home every month and denies any masses or lumps in the breasts or axilla.

Review of Systems

The patient's ROS is positive for skin "rash" to left breast, increased warmth and pain in the affected area, pain in the left shoulder, and limited ROM due to "tightness." Her ROS is negative for fever, chills, weight loss, breast lumps, vomiting, headache, weakness, abdominal pain, cough, SOB, chest wall pain, acid reflux, easy bruising or bleeding, and bone or joint pain.

Relevant History

The patient's medical history is unremarkable, without any diagnosed adult illnesses. She is up to date on all vaccinations. She has never had surgery but had two overnight hospitalizations for the birth of her sons. Her last physical exam was 7 months ago and included routine labs for anemia and cholesterol, which were normal. She was referred for mammogram and colonoscopy at that time but has not yet scheduled these tests. She is in menopause. She has been married to her female partner for the past 18 years and is happy in her relationship. She and her partner are sexually active in a monogamous relationship and she had no previous sexual partners prior to this relationship. She was tested for all STIs, including HIV, about 10 years ago, all of which were negative.

Allergies

No known drug allergies; no known food allergies.

Medications

- Famotidine 20 mg QD PRN for heartburn.
- Vitamin B_{12} QD.

PHYSICAL EXAMINATION

- *Vitals:* T 37.5°C (99.5°F), P 90, R 14, BP 118/78, HT 165 cm (64 in.), WT 60.7 kg (134 lb), BMI 23.0.
- *General:* Nervous-appearing female, mildly uncomfortable but nontoxic appearing.
- *Psychiatric:* Appears nervous and worried but calm and cooperative.
- *Skin, Hair, and Nails:* General skin exam reveals dark brown color (Fitzpatrick V), unremarkable except for a small keloid scar on her right thigh and a few scattered skin tags on her superior aspect of upper back/superior shoulder areas. Large patch-like area of violaceous/pink skin on dark brown skin tone, dimpled and rough in texture on left breast 1 cm from areola, circumferential to areola and extending to mid-breast with tenderness to palpation and increased warmth and pitting. No induration or drainage from the lesion or nipple. Right breast without skin changes. No abnormal findings with hair or nails.
- *ENT/Mouth:* Nares patent, oropharynx clear.
- *Neck:* No cervical/supraclavicular/occipital lymphadenopathy. No nodules or lumps palpable.
- *Breasts:* Pendulous breasts BL, with asymmetry of the left breast resting more superficial to the right breast. Skin as noted previously. No palpable lumps or masses in either breast. Nipples without deformity or drainage. Left breast tender to palpation over affected violaceous/pink area with large area of induration near areola. No palpable lymphadenopathy in BL axilla.
- *Lungs:* CTA bilaterally without wheezes/rhonchi/crackles.
- *Heart:* RRR without murmur.
- *Abdomen:* Soft, nontender, not distended, active BS throughout.
- *Musculoskeletal:* Limited flexion and abduction of left shoulder due to tightness referred from the left breast with active ROM. FROM passively on left shoulder.
- *Neurologic:* A&O×3, CN II to XII intact.

CLINICAL DISCUSSION QUESTIONS

1. What is the differential diagnosis?

____

____

____

____

2. What is the most likely diagnosis? Why?

____

____

____

____

3. Demonstrate your understanding about the pathophysiology of the most likely diagnosis.

____

____

____

____

4. Should tests/imaging studies be ordered? Which ones? Why? Think about tests/imaging beyond the primary care setting as well.

5. What are the next appropriate steps in management?

6. What are the diagnostic challenges, diagnostic studies, and disparities in race and socioeconomic factors of the diagnosis? Provide references for your response.

7. What are the pertinent ICD-10 and CPT (E/M) codes for this visit? Provide a short rationale.

8. What is the appropriate patient education topic for this case?

9. If not managed appropriately, what is/are the medical/legal concern(s) that may arise?

10. Think about interprofessional collaboration for this case. Provide a list of specialties or other disciplines and indicate what contribution these professionals might make to managing the patient.

BEDSIDE MANNER QUESTIONS

11. What would your communication style/approach be with this patient?

12. If the patient shows distress at what you communicate, how would you provide support?

Answers available at courseconnect.springerpub.com.

CASE 44

BLOOD IN STOOL, ADULT FEMALE

Chief Complaint

"Blood in stool."

History of Present Illness

A 52-year-old woman with obesity and hypothyroidism presents to an urgent care clinic affiliated with her PCP's practice for rectal bleeding for the past 4 months. Initially, it happened about once a week during a bowel movement but was currently occurring daily with all bowel movements. She describes the blood as approximately 1 teaspoon, dark red, and mixed in the stool. She denies any associated rectal or abdominal pain, and her bowel movements are regular every day without change, although they do seem thinner, which she attributes to starting a low-carbohydrate diet 4 months ago. She relays a history of internal hemorrhoids after the birth of her daughter 20 years ago, with rare bleeding throughout the years that always improves within a day of applying OTC hemorrhoid cream. Despite using this cream daily now, there has been no improvement in current symptoms. Though she was referred for colonoscopy screening at age 50, she never scheduled it because she was "afraid of the prep" and did not want to miss a whole day of work. She states she called her regular PCP 3 months ago about her bleeding. "He told to me that my insurance allows me to see the gastroenterologist without a referral, so I should go there and get a colonoscopy done." The procedure is scheduled in 3 weeks, the earliest available for the "routine screening" referral sent. The patient asked whether "the take-home test" or a "virtual colonoscopy" could be ordered today for quicker results.

Review of Systems

The patient endorses fatigue and weight loss of 12 lb in 4 months, which she attributes to dieting, and occasional night sweats, which she attributes to menopause. She denies fever or chills. She endorses increasing SOB when walking upstairs or hills for the past month but denies any chest pain, palpitations, or syncope; endorses dizziness when standing up quickly but denies headache, weakness, or paresthesia; denies cough, wheezing, or hemoptysis; denies anorexia, heartburn, nausea/vomiting, diarrhea, or melena; denies any dysuria, hematuria, vaginal bleeding or discharge, or pelvic pain; denies any increased bruising or swollen lymph nodes; denies any skin rashes, lesions, or itching; and denies insomnia, anxiety, or depression.

Relevant History

- The patient has struggled with obesity since her pregnancy at age 32, after which she was diagnosed with hypothyroidism. She has taken levothyroxine 112 mcg QD for 20 years but takes no other medications or supplements. She has no prior history of heart, lung, GI, or bleeding disorders, and she has no prior surgeries or hospitalizations.
- Her parents are alive and healthy in their late 70s; she believes her maternal grandmother died in her 60s of "some kind of stomach cancer." There is no family history of heart disease, DM, or bleeding disorder.
- She is married and sexually active. She does not smoke or use any recreational drugs. She drinks 2 glasses of wine every night with dinner.

Allergies

None.

MEDICATIONS

Levothyroxine 112 mcg QD.

PHYSICAL EXAMINATION

- *Vitals:* T 37.2°C (99.0°F), P 98, R 18, BP 110/62, SPo_2 97%, HT 157.5 cm (62 in.), WT 91.2 kg (201 lb), BMI 36.0.
- *General:* Well-developed, obese Caucasian female; A&O; all vital signs stable; in no acute distress.
- *Psychiatric:* Broad affect euthymic mood, fluent speech, average insight.
- *Skin, Hair, and Nails:* Warm and dry, pallor of skin noted, nail beds, and conjunctivae. No jaundice or rashes present. No abnormal findings with hair or nails.
- *Lungs:* CTA bilaterally with no adventitious sounds. Good effort with no accessory muscle use.
- *Heart:* RRR with no murmurs, gallops, or rubs.
- *Abdomen:* Protuberant noted with central obesity. NABS in all quadrants with no bruits noted. Soft, nontender, nondistended; no masses, organomegaly, or hernia present.
- *Genital/Rectal:* Genital exam deferred; rectal exam shows normal sphincter tone, no fissures noted, visible small nontender nonthrombosed external hemorrhoid visible at 6 o'clock, and a small nontender internal hemorrhoid at 9 o'clock. Brown hard stool and gross blood noted in vault, which is guaiac FOBT positive.
- *Extremities:* No edema, clubbing, or cyanosis. Radial and dorsalis pedis pulses 2+ bilaterally.
- *Neurologic:* Gait steady; no tremors, no focal deficits.

CLINICAL DISCUSSION QUESTIONS

1. What is the differential diagnosis?

2. What is the most likely diagnosis? Why?

3. Demonstrate your understanding about the pathophysiology of the most likely diagnosis.

4. Should tests/imaging studies be ordered? Which ones? Why? Think about tests/imaging beyond the primary care setting as well.

5. What are the next appropriate steps in management?

6. What are the incidence and screening recommendations for this diagnosis? Provide references for your response.

7. What are the pertinent ICD-10 and CPT (E/M) codes for this visit? Provide a short rationale.

8. What is the appropriate patient education topic for this case?

9. If not managed appropriately, what is/are the medical/legal concern(s) that may arise?

10. Think about interprofessional collaboration for this case. Provide a list of specialties or other disciplines and indicate what contribution these professionals might make to managing the patient.

BEDSIDE MANNER QUESTION

11. What would your communication style/approach be with this patient?

Answers available at courseconnect.springerpub.com

ERECTION DIFFICULTIES, ADULT MALE

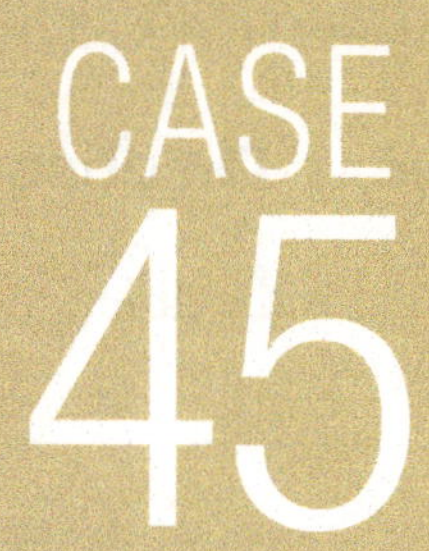

Chief Complaint

"Erection difficulties."

History of Present Illness

A 23-year-old cisgender man presents to his PCP with a 7-day history of inability to have an erection. He states this has never happened before. The patient had sex with a partner the night before his symptoms started and was fine. He denies any trauma to his penis or any pain during sexual activity. He has talked to his friends about it and was told it was probably stress related. He reports infrequent marijuana use and 2 nights weekly of drinking, 6 drinks a night. He has been smoking two to three cigarettes per day for the last 3 years. He does not believe the erection difficulties occurred because of alcohol or marijuana use. The patient reports he gets enough sleep. He reports no changes in urinary function or flow. He denies any rectal pain or pressure. He states he still has morning erections but not as hard as usual. He denies changes in his interest in or response to sexual arousal. He does report significant life stress from school and exams and has a history of depression. He denies any previous STI testing or diagnosis but would like to be tested and reports a total of three to four male partners in his lifetime. The patient engages in receptive anal intercourse (condoms sometimes) and oral sex with no condoms. His last sexual contact was 8 days ago, when he had receptive anal intercourse with no condom.

Review of Systems

The patient's ROS is positive for erectile dysfunction and stress. His ROS is negative for lack of appetite, lack of energy, lack of concentration, anxiety, fever, chills, dysuria, urinary urgency, hematuria, penile discharge, rash, SOB, or chest pain.

Relevant History

The patient has a history of depression and attention deficit disorder. He is a graduate student in architecture. No significant family medical history.

Allergies

No known drug allergies; no known food allergies.

Medications

None.

Physical Examination

- *Vitals:* T 36.4°C (97.6°F), P 69, R 16, BP 112/70, HT 170 cm (67 in.), WT 60.3 kg (133 lb), BMI 20.8.
- *General:* Vital signs stable, no acute distress.
- *Psychiatric:* Engaged but distant (not comfortable talking about this today). Appears anxious.
- *Genital/Rectal:* Rectal exam deferred. GU exam revealed healthy-appearing circumcised penis. No edema, discharge, or erythema. There were also no ulcers or lesions. Chaperone for this exam was offered and declined by patient.

CLINICAL DISCUSSION QUESTIONS

1. What is the differential diagnosis?

2. What is the most likely diagnosis? Why?

3. Demonstrate your understanding about the pathophysiology of the most likely diagnosis.

4. Should tests/imaging studies be ordered? Which ones? Why? Think about tests/imaging beyond the primary care setting as well.

5. What are the next appropriate steps in management?

6. What are the prevalence and contributing factors of this diagnosis in young adult males? What is a first-line recommendation to help treat this condition without medication? Provide references for your answers.

7. What are the pertinent ICD-10 and CPT (E/M) codes for this visit? Provide a short rationale.

8. What is the appropriate patient education topic for this case?

9. If not managed appropriately, what is/are the medical/legal concern(s) that may arise?

10. Think about interprofessional collaboration for this case. Provide a list of specialties or other disciplines and indicate what contribution these professionals might make to managing the patient.

Bedside Manner Question

11. What would your communication style/approach be with this patient?

Answers available at courseconnect.springerpub.com.

CASE 46

UNEXPLAINED WEIGHT GAIN, ADULT FEMALE

Chief Complaint

"Unexplained weight gain."

History of Present Illness

A 34-year-old Caucasian woman presents to her PCP with a 1-year history of weight gain despite efforts to eat healthy and increase physical activity. She is married and a mother of three children, 13-year-old twin boys and a 6-year-old girl. She states she did not pay attention to the gradual weight gain until about 4 months ago, when she began making efforts to lose weight to include walking and eating less fast food.

Review of Systems

The patient's ROS is positive for a 25-lb weight gain over the past year. Her last menstrual period was 2 weeks ago. Her ROS is negative for fatigue, dry skin, acne, fever, thinning hair, HTN, swelling, weakness, reduced exercise tolerance, abdominal pain or distension, constipation, excessive hair growth, nipple discharge, anxiety, depression, substance abuse concerns, cold intolerance, difficulty sleeping, snoring, joint pain, polydipsia, or polyuria.

Relevant History

The patient's relevant history includes vitamin D deficiency. She smokes half a pack of cigarettes per day. The patient admits she is less active than she used to be and consumes a diet high in carbohydrates. She denies alcohol or illicit drug use. She lives with her husband and describes it as stressful. Her family history is positive for T2DM, HTN, hyperlipidemia, and early heart disease.

Allergies

No known drug allergies; no known food allergies.

Medications

- OTC multivitamin QD.
- Vitamin D 50,000 IU weekly.

Physical Examination

- *Vitals:* T 36.7°C (98.1°F), P 70, R 18, BP 116/77, HT 170 cm (67 in.), WT 93 kg (205 lb), BMI 32.1.
- *General:* Obese and well groomed in no acute distress.
- *Psychiatric:* Normal mood and affect.
- *Skin, Hair, and Nails:* Skin warm and dry with no excessive facial hair or rash. No abnormal findings with nails.
- *Neck:* Thyroid is normal size; consistency and is nontender.
- *Lungs:* CTA bilaterally.
- *Heart:* RRR, radial pulse 2+ bilaterally.
- *Lymphatic:* Nonpalpable cervical nodes

- *Abdomen:* Rounded, nondistended, soft, nontender, normal BS.
- *Musculoskeletal:* No extremity edema. FROM both UE and LE, BL.
- *Neurologic:* A&O×3 without tics or tremors.

Clinical Discussion Questions

1. What is the differential diagnosis?

2. What is the most likely diagnosis? Why?

3. Demonstrate your understanding about the pathophysiology of the most likely diagnosis.

4. Should tests/imaging studies be ordered? Which ones? Why? Think about tests/imaging beyond the primary care setting as well.

5. What are the next appropriate steps in management?

6. What are the diagnostic criteria and risk factors for this diagnosis? Provide references for your response.

7. What are the pertinent ICD-10 and CPT (E/M) codes for this visit? Provide a short rationale.

8. What is the appropriate patient education topic for this case?

9. If not managed appropriately, what is/are the medical/legal concern(s) that may arise?

10. Think about interprofessional collaboration for this case. Provide a list of specialties or other disciplines and indicate what contribution these professionals might make to managing the patient.

BEDSIDE MANNER QUESTIONS

11. What would your communication style/approach be with this patient?

12. If the patient shows distress at what you communicate, how would you provide support?

Answers available at courseconnect.springerpub.com.

CASE 47

WORSENING, SHARP ABDOMINAL PAIN, ADULT FEMALE

Chief Complaint

"Worsening, sharp abdominal pain."

History of Present Illness

A 22-year-old woman presents as a new patient to the primary care clinic, complaining of abdominal pain for the past week and a half. The pain became worse while having sexual intercourse with her boyfriend today. She states she had intercourse around 2.5 hours prior to arrival. She describes the pain as sharp in nature, located in the suprapubic region, rated 8/10, and constant; but it does not radiate, although she also has lower back pain. Her last menstrual period was almost 3 weeks ago. Her cycles are noted to be regular and last approximately 3 days. She states she has never experienced this type of pain before. The pain is exacerbated by movement and sexual intercourse, and she denies any relieving factors. She states she is currently in a monogamous relationship with her boyfriend of 2 years, and they do not use any form of contraception.

Review of Systems

The patient's ROS is positive for suprapubic pain, low back pain, dyspareunia, nausea, fever, chills, frequency, and yellow-white vaginal discharge. The ROS is negative for vomiting, diarrhea, urgency, dysuria, anorexia, chest pain, SOB, headaches, dizziness, and abnormal vaginal bleeding.

Relevant History

The patient is a full-time graduate student who lives alone. She has never been pregnant, denies tobacco use, drinks a glass of wine socially approximately two to three times a month, and denies recreational drug use. She has a history of trichomonas diagnosed and treated at age 18.

Allergies

No known drug allergies; no known food allergies.

Medications

OTC multivitamin QD.

Physical Examination

- *Vitals:* T 37.7°C (99.9°F), P 67, R 18, BP 127/86, SpO_2 98%, HT 167.64 cm (66 in.), WT 90.72 kg (200 lb), BMI 32.27.
- *General:* Ill-appearing obese female lying in the right lateral decubitus position, in moderate distress secondary to pain.
- *Skin, Hair, and Nails:* No visible rash; no abnormal findings on hair or nails.
- *Psychiatric:* Cooperative, slightly anxious, likely secondary to pain.
- *Chest:* Normal anteroposterior diameter, symmetric chest wall expansion, no chest wall tenderness to palpation.
- *Lungs:* Breath sounds CTA bilaterally, without wheezing, rales, or rhonchi.
- *Heart:* RRR, S1, S2, no murmurs, rubs, or gallops.

- *Abdomen:* Nondistended, NABS, soft, tenderness noted in the RLQ, no guarding, no rebound, no masses appreciated; psoas, Rovsing, and obturator signs all negative.
- *Genital/Rectal:* Normal external genitalia without rash, ulcerations, nodularities, or abnormal lesions. Speculum exam notes moist, pink, vaginal walls with mild erythema, frothy, thin, yellow-white discharge pooled in the posterior fornix noted; no lesions or ulcerations. Cervix is erythematous, with noted discharge. Cervical motion tenderness noted. Bimanual exam notes positive bilateral adnexal tenderness to palpation, with no palpable masses appreciated. Rectal exam notes no lesions or ulcerations, normal sphincter tone, not tender to palpation. No palpable inguinal lymphadenopathy. Genital/rectal exam was performed with a chaperone (MA) present in the room.
- *Musculoskeletal:* Negative BL costovertebral angle tenderness.
- *Neurologic:* A&O×3. CN II to XII grossly intact.

Clinical Discussion Questions

1. What is the differential diagnosis?

2. What is the most likely diagnosis? Why?

3. Demonstrate your understanding about the pathophysiology of the most likely diagnosis.

4. Should tests/imaging studies be ordered? Which ones? Why? Think about tests/imaging beyond the primary care setting as well.

5. What are the next appropriate steps in management?

6. What are the adverse outcomes and treatment recommendations for this diagnosis and its relationship to trichomonas? List the name of your references.

7. What are the pertinent ICD-10 and CPT (E/M) codes for this visit? Provide a short rationale.

8. What is the appropriate patient education topic for this case?

9. If not managed appropriately, what is/are the medical/legal concern(s) that may arise?

10. Think about interprofessional collaboration for this case. Provide a list of specialties or other disciplines and indicate what contribution these professionals might make to managing the patient.

BEDSIDE MANNER QUESTION

11. What would your communication style/approach be with this patient?

Answers available at courseconnect.springerpub.com.

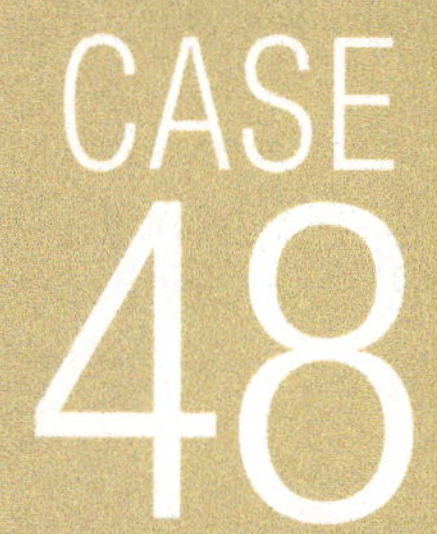

LUMP IN BREAST, ADULT MALE

Chief Complaint

"Lump in breast."

History of Present Illness

A 42-year-old, generally healthy man presents for evaluation of a mass on his right chest wall/breast. He states he has a "hard nodule" below his right nipple that he noticed 2 days ago; it is not painful and has not changed. He denies trauma or injury to the area. He reports no galactorrhea or bleeding from the nipple or skin and no skin changes on the chest. He denies any masses anywhere else on his body. He denies any systemic symptoms such as weight changes, fevers, or night sweats. He has never had anything like this before; nothing makes it better or worse, and he has not tried any medication or treatment at this time.

Review of Systems

The ROS is positive for breast mass and a history of moderate erectile dysfunction after a vascular injury to his penis several years ago, and he states his erectile dysfunction may have worsened recently. The ROS is negative for skin lesions; chills or sweats; fatigue, malaise, or weakness; polyuria; polydipsia; polyphagia; heat or cold intolerance; change in voice, hair, or skin; excessive sweating or weight change; easy bruising or bleeding; abdominal pain; early satiety; changes in appetite or bowel habits; dysuria; obstructive voiding symptoms; testicular pain; swelling or testicular mass; or urethral discharge.

Relevant History

The patient's medical history is significant for carcinoma of the thyroid, with a total thyroidectomy and radiation treatment (age 16); traumatic vascular injury to penis/urethra with subsequent scarring, resulting in erectile dysfunction (age 22); and vasectomy without complications (age 40). His social history includes alcohol use (4 drinks/week), no tobacco use, and regular exercise. He is a firefighter, married with one child (age 7). His family history is significant for bladder cancer in father (age 56), breast cancer in paternal grandmother (age 59), ovarian cancer in a paternal aunt (age 43), lung cancer in maternal grandmother (age 75), and bone cancer in his maternal grandfather (age 55).

Allergies

No known drug allergies; no known food allergies.

Medications

- Levothyroxine 175 mcg QD.
- Sildenafil 25 mg PRN.

Physical Examination

- *Vitals:* T 37°C (98.6°F), P 54, R 16, BP 140/83; HT 178 cm (70 in.), WT 70 kg (155 lb), BMI 22.
- *General:* Well-developed, well-nourished male in no apparent distress; appears fit; appears stated age.
- *Neck:* Faint thyroidectomy scar across the anterior neck; no palpable thyroid tissue or neck mass noted; no cervical adenopathy or tenderness bilaterally.
- *Lungs:* CTA bilaterally without wheezes, rales, or rhonchi.

- *Breast:* Right-sided retro-areolar nontender breast mass palpated, firm, smooth, and mobile, approximately 3 cm in diameter without skin changes or retraction of the nipple; no erythema or warmth; no galactorrhea; left breast with no abnormal findings; no axillary or supraclavicular adenopathy bilaterally.
- *Heart:* RRR without murmur, rubs, or gallops.
- *Abdomen:* Soft, flat, nontender; positive BS; no masses, no hepatosplenomegaly.
- *Genital/Rectal:* Circumcised penis with midline urethra; no plaques, no urethral discharge; scrotum without swelling or tenderness; testes palpated without masses or tenderness bilaterally. Rectal exam deferred.

CLINICAL DISCUSSION QUESTIONS

1. What is the differential diagnosis?

2. What is the most likely diagnosis? Why?

3. Demonstrate your understanding about the pathophysiology of the most likely diagnosis.

4. Should tests/imaging studies be ordered? Which ones? Why? Think about tests/imaging beyond the primary care setting as well.

5. What are the next appropriate steps in management?

6. What are the causes of this diagnosis and the most helpful diagnostic imaging studies for the initial workup? Why thorough follow-up is vital for this diagnosis? Provide references for your response.

7. What are the pertinent ICD-10 and CPT (E/M) codes for this visit? Provide a short rationale.

8. What is the appropriate patient education topic for this case?

9. If not managed appropriately, what is/are the medical/legal concern(s) that may arise?

10. Think about interprofessional collaboration for this case. Provide a list of specialties or other disciplines and indicate what contribution these professionals might make to managing the patient.

Bedside Manner Questions

11. What would your communication style/approach be with this patient?

12. If a patient is distressed by the diagnosis, what might offer support?

Answers available at courseconnect.springerpub.com.

FREQUENT ILLNESS AND FATIGUE, ADULT FEMALE

CASE 49

Chief Complaint

"Frequent illness and fatigue."

History of Present Illness

A 34-year-old African American woman presents for a third time in 6 months complaining of upper respiratory symptoms. At this time, her symptoms, including cough, are resolving. She reports that she tends to get sick easily. She is less concerned about her current symptoms but more concerned about always getting sick. Three months ago, she was also diagnosed with community-acquired pneumonia. Over the past 3 months, she has noted marked fatigue and generalized achiness. Nothing seems to help with her symptoms. She has taken ibuprofen for her symptoms with fair relief. She does not eat a well-balanced diet and calls her diet "the typical American diet."

Review of Systems

The patient's ROS is positive for fatigue, generalized myalgias, and a nonproductive resolving cough. She denies recent changes in weight or appetite, heart palpitation, SOB, pale skin (pallor), heat or cold intolerance, nausea, vomiting, diarrhea, constipation, polyuria, polydipsia, polyphagia, headache, dizziness, numbness, and tingling in UE or LE. She also denies fever, chills, and chest pain. She denies anxiety and depression.

Relevant History

Her history is positive for being overweight. She was treated for pneumonia 3 months ago. Her immunizations are up to date. Her surgical history includes a Cesarean section in 2015. She has no hospitalizations outside of childbirth. She was tested for HIV 9 months ago and the result was negative. Her last physical exam was 9 months ago. She has no history of cancer, DM, HTN, or thyroid problems. The patient is married and has two young children. Her marriage is monogamous, and she has been married for 10 years. Her husband had vasectomy a few years ago. She is a kindergarten teacher. She reports missing work at least twice a month due to illness and fatigue. She does not use alcohol, illicit drugs, or tobacco products. She is not physically active and does not spend much time outside. Her family history is noncontributory.

Allergies

Penicillin (hives); no known food allergies.

Medications

None.

Physical Examination

- *Vitals:* T 36.94°C (98.5°F), P 86, R 16, BP 134/72, WT 68 kg (150 lb) HT 160 cm (63 in.), BMI 26.6.
- *General:* Well nourished, well developed, in no acute distress. Overweight.
- *Psychiatric:* Calm and cooperative.

- *Skin, Hair, and Nails:* Skin warm and without rash; no pallor of skin; no abnormal findings on hair and nails.
- *Head:* Normocephalic; no deformities noted.
- *Eyes:* PERRLA.
- *ENT/Mouth:* TM clear bilaterally; no pharyngeal erythema; no nasal deformity.
- *Neck:* Supple; no thyromegaly; FROM.
- *Lungs:* CTA in all lung fields; no wheezing; no crackles.
- *Heart:* RRR, no murmurs or gallops noted.
- *Musculoskeletal:* FROM in all extremities; no muscle tenderness with palpation; no edema or deformities noted.
- *Neurologic:* A&O×3; follows commands; CN II to XII grossly intact.

Clinical Discussion Questions

1. What is the differential diagnosis?

2. What is the most likely diagnosis? Why?

3. Demonstrate your understanding about the pathophysiology of the most likely diagnosis.

4. Should tests/imaging studies be ordered? Which ones? Why? Think about tests/imaging beyond the primary care setting as well.

5. What are the next appropriate steps in management?

6. What are the risk factors and treatment approach of the diagnosis? Provide references for your responses.

7. What are the pertinent ICD-10 and CPT (E/M) codes for this visit? Provide a short rationale.

8. What is the appropriate patient education topic for this case?

9. If not managed appropriately, what is/are the medical/legal concern(s) that may arise?

10. Think about interprofessional collaboration for this case. Provide a list of specialties or other disciplines and indicate what contribution these professionals might make to managing the patient.

BEDSIDE MANNER QUESTION

11. What would your communication style/approach be with this patient?

Answers available at courseconnect.springerpub.com.

PAINFUL URINATION, ADOLESCENT MALE

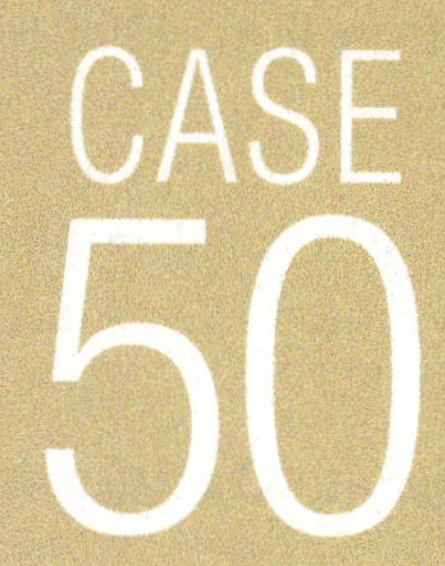

Chief Complaint

"Burning sensation while urinating."

History of Present Illness

A 17-year-old male with no significant medical history presents with a complaint of urinary symptoms. He reports that for the last week, he has noticed mild burning with urination. He has noticed a thick and white/yellow penile discharge. He states he had unprotected sex with a new partner about 2 weeks ago. His partner is asymptomatic. He has not been tested for STIs in the past and says he does not consistently use protection. He has had four sexual partners in the last 2 years and claims his last sexual encounter was unprotected. He has noticed slight testicular discomfort, with 2/10 pain. He is concerned about these symptoms and asking about what he could have. He denies fever and genital lesions.

Review of Systems

The patient's ROS is positive for dysuria, penile discharge, and testicular pain. The ROS is negative for fever, recent illnesses, chest pain, SOB, abdominal pain, diarrhea, constipation, nausea, vomiting, and mood change.

Relevant History

The patient is a senior in high school with no known medical problems or surgical history. His immunizations are up to date. He denies regular tobacco use but has vaped a few times. He drinks alcohol at parties maybe once every 1 to 2 months. He experimented with marijuana once but denies other illicit drug usage. He works at a department store at the local mall.

Allergies

No known drug allergies; no known food allergies.

Medications

None.

Physical Examination

- *Vitals:* T 36.5°C (97.8°F), P 103, R 20, BP 115/78, HT 172.7 cm (68 in.), WT 71.7 kg (158 lb), BMI 24.
- *General:* No acute distress.
- *Psychiatric:* Normal affect. Responds to questions appropriately.
- *Skin, Hair, and Nails:* No rashes or skin lesions visible. No abnormal findings with hair or nails.
- *Head:* Normocephalic, atraumatic.
- *Chest:* No labored breathing, chest symmetrical.
- *Lungs:* CTA bilaterally; no wheezing, rhonchi, or rales.
- *Heart:* Mild tachycardia, no murmur appreciated.
- *Abdomen:* Nontender, nondistended, normal BS.

- *Genital/Rectal:* Uncircumcised penis, no skin lesions. Mild tenderness to epididymis on right side, scant white discharge from urethra.
- *Neurologic:* No focal deficits.

CLINICAL DISCUSSION QUESTIONS

1. What is the differential diagnosis?

2. What is the most likely diagnosis? Why?

3. Demonstrate your understanding about the pathophysiology of the most likely diagnosis.

4. Should tests/imaging studies be ordered? Which ones? Why? Think about tests/imaging beyond the primary care setting as well.

5. What are the next appropriate steps in management?

6. What are the incidence, treatment options, and treatment approach for this diagnosis? Provide references for your response.

7. What are the pertinent ICD-10 and CPT (E/M) codes for this visit? Provide a short rationale.

8. What is the appropriate patient education topic for this case?

9. If not managed appropriately, what is/are the medical/legal concern(s) that may arise?

10. Think about interprofessional collaboration for this case. Provide a list of specialties or other disciplines and indicate what contribution these professionals might make to managing the patient.

BEDSIDE MANNER QUESTION

11. What would your communication style/approach be with this patient?

Answers available at courseconnect.springerpub.com.

COUGHING AND WHEEZING, PEDIATRIC MALE

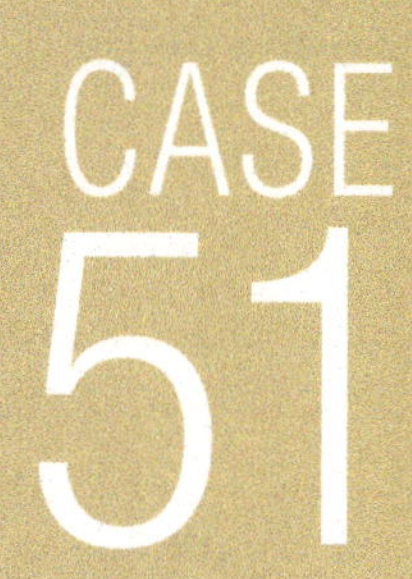

Chief Complaint

"Coughing and wheezing."

History of Present Illness

A 6-year-old boy presents with his mother to a new PCP with a 6-week history of coughing and wheezing. He has not had routine well-child checks due to several relocations, but he is up to date on vaccines and his mother would like to establish care. His mother says the coughing and wheezing have been steadily worsening over the past several weeks during winter season but have been significantly worse in the past 2 weeks. He coughs throughout the daytime and wakes up several times at night during the week. In the past week, he has used his albuterol inhaler QD for cough/wheeze, and sometimes it is so bad that he "can't breathe." He has gone to the ED twice in the past year for coughing and wheezing; was given nebulized breathing treatments with significant improvement of symptoms; and was subsequently discharged home with an albuterol inhaler, 5 days of oral steroids, and instructions to follow up with the PCP. He has never required hospitalization. His mother says he is a very active child and loves to play soccer, but in the past 2 weeks, he has not been able to keep up with his teammates due to difficulty breathing while playing.

Review of Systems

ROS is positive for dry chronic cough, SOB, and wheezing. The ROS is negative for fever, eye redness or discharge, nasal congestion/discharge, sneezing, earache, sore throat, decreased intake, decreased energy, decreased voids, change in stools, bulky/greasy stools, weight loss, night sweats, or rash.

Relevant History

The patient's past medical history is unremarkable except for the coughing and wheezing. There is no history of pneumonia, recurrent infections, seasonal allergies, or food allergies. TB skin test prior to starting kindergarten was negative last year. His mother smoked cigarettes during her pregnancy with this child and throughout his childhood until the present. He is in the first grade and has average performance, but he seems more distracted and impulsive in the past 2 months at school. He lives at home in an apartment with his mother and two older siblings (no pets). Parents had an amicable divorce 3 months ago and the patient sees his father every other weekend. Mother continues to smoke cigarettes but "only outside." Family history is significant for biologic father with asthma as a child.

Allergies

No known drug allergies; no known food allergies.

Medications

Albuterol inhaler 2 puffs every 4 to 6 hours PRN.

Physical Examination

- *Vitals:* T 37.1°C (98.8°F), P 100, RR 24, BP 110/70, SpO_2 97%, WT 22.7 kg (50 lb), 75th percentile; HT 120 cm (47 in.), 75th percentile; BMI 15.8, 63rd percentile.
- *General:* Well-appearing, no acute distress, answering questions in complete sentences, talkative.

- *Skin, Hair, and Nails:* Normal skin turgor, no rashes or dry patches. No abnormal findings with hair or nails.
- *Head:* Normocephalic/atraumatic.
- *Eyes:* EOM intact bilaterally, PERRLA bilaterally, no scleral injection, no eye discharge.
- *ENT:* TMs normal bilaterally. Normal nasal turbinates bilaterally with pink mucosa, no discharge, normal pharynx. 2+ tonsils bilaterally without erythema, edema, or exudate.
- *Chest:* Mild barrel chest, no retractions.
- *Lungs:* End-expiratory wheeze diffusely in all anterior and posterior lung fields bilaterally, decreased air movement throughout.
- *Heart:* RRR without murmur.

CLINICAL DISCUSSION QUESTIONS

1. What is the differential diagnosis?

2. What is the most likely diagnosis? Why?

3. Demonstrate an understanding about the pathophysiology of the most likely diagnosis.

4. Should tests/imaging studies be ordered? Which ones? Why? Think about tests/imaging beyond the primary care setting as well.

5. What are the next appropriate steps in management?

6. What are the risk factors, diagnostic studies, efficacy of medications, and medical costs associated with the diagnosis? Provide references for your responses.

7. What are the pertinent ICD-10 and CPT (E/M) codes for this visit? Provide a short rationale.

8. What is the appropriate patient education topic for this case?

9. If not managed appropriately, what is/are the medical/legal concern(s) that may arise?

10. Think about interprofessional collaboration for this case. Provide a list of specialties or other disciplines and indicate what contribution these professionals might make to managing the patient.

Bedside Manner Question

11. What would your communication style/approach be with this patient and his mother?

Answers available at courseconnect.springerpub.com.

CASE 52

CONSTIPATION, ADOLESCENT FEMALE

Chief Complaint

"Constipation."

History of Present Illness

A 17-year-old young woman presents to her PCP with complaints of persistent constipation for about 6 months. Her mother is present and confirms her daughter often complains of feeling full after just a few bites of food, experiences abdominal discomfort and bloating, and has difficulty passing bowel movements. The patient admits she does not always drink enough water through her day but eats a balanced diet and tries to stay active. Her mother reports having tried polyethylene glycol for her daughter "a few times" with some benefit, but no other interventions have been attempted. On further discussion, the patient does admit that it has been harder for her to be active lately as she always feels tired. She is a runner and a swimmer but notes her performance in both sports has declined and she feels "slow" and "blah" most days. Her mother reports she sleeps about 7 to 8 hours per night, does not recall her snoring or gasping for breath, and denies hearing her wake often at night. The patient denies being overly anxious or depressed and reports good social activity. She is doing well in school, behaves appropriately at home, and works part-time at a pizzeria with good work behaviors. Her only other concern is a 7-lb weight gain over the past few months despite having decreased appetite but states, "I just thought it was because I wasn't going to the bathroom enough."

Review of Systems

The patient's ROS is positive for constipation, abdominal discomfort and bloating, weight gain, and fatigue. Her ROS is negative for vomiting or diarrhea, blood in stools, fever, and chills. She denies changes in her menstrual cycle. Her ROS is negative for chest pain or palpitations, SOB, dizziness or headache, and anxiety or depression. No hair or skin changes are noted, as well as no joint pain or swelling.

Relevant History

The patient had a fracture of fifth metatarsal of the right foot at age 12; her last menstrual period was 2 weeks ago. She attends 11th grade in a public school, with As and Bs in all classes. She denies smoking (including vaping), drinking, or alcohol use. She lives at home with her mother and a younger brother. Parents are divorced but her father is very active in her life and supportive. She denies sexual activity and has no history of STIs. Her vaccinations and preventive screening are up to date and unremarkable. Her family history is significant for mother with hypothyroidism and paternal grandfather with T2DM.

Allergies

No known drug allergies; no known food allergies.

Medications

Polyethylene glycol 3350 PRN.

PHYSICAL EXAMINATION

- *Vitals:* T 36°C (96.8°F); P 68; R 14; BP 108/64; WT 68 kg (150 lb), increased from 65 kg (143 lb) last visit 3 months ago; HT 157.5 cm (62 in.); BMI 24.2.
- *General:* A&O×3, well groomed.
- *Psychiatric:* Normal affect, pleasant, and cooperative.
- *Skin, Hair, and Nails:* Skin dry but without rash or lesions. No abnormal findings with hair or nails.
- *Neck:* Supple with some mild thyromegaly, no nodules. No cervical lymph nodes.
- *Lungs:* CTA with normal respiratory effort.
- *Heart:* S1 S2 RRR; no murmur noted.
- *Abdomen:* Mild distention with firmness and mild tenderness on palpation. Stool detected in descending colon.
- *Rectal:* Hard stool in rectal vault noted but no blood. No internal or external hemorrhoids; negative for occult blood.
- *Musculoskeletal:* No redness or swelling of joints, with FROM.
- *Neurologic:* Patellar DTRs 1+ bilaterally (mildly diminished), normal gait and station. CN grossly intact.

CLINICAL DISCUSSION QUESTIONS

1. What is the differential diagnosis?

____

____

____

____

2. What is the most likely diagnosis? Why?

____

____

____

____

3. Demonstrate your understanding about the pathophysiology of the most likely diagnosis.

____

____

____

____

4. Should tests/imaging studies be ordered? Which ones? Why? Think about tests/imaging beyond the primary care setting as well.

5. What are the next appropriate steps in management?

6. What are the different types of organ dysfunction (primary organ associated with the case) and what is the role of autoimmune diseases of this diagnosis? Provide references for your responses.

7. What are the pertinent ICD-10 and CPT (E/M) codes for this visit? Provide a short rationale.

8. What is the appropriate patient education topic for this case?

9. If not managed appropriately, what is/are the medical/legal concern(s) that may arise?

10. Think about interprofessional collaboration for this case. Provide a list of specialties or other disciplines and indicate what contribution these professionals might make to managing the patient.

BEDSIDE MANNER QUESTIONS

11. What would be your communication style/approach with this patient and her mother?

12. If the patient and her mother are distressed by a diagnosis, what might offer support?

Answers available at courseconnect.springerpub.com.

ABDOMINAL PAIN, ADOLESCENT MALE

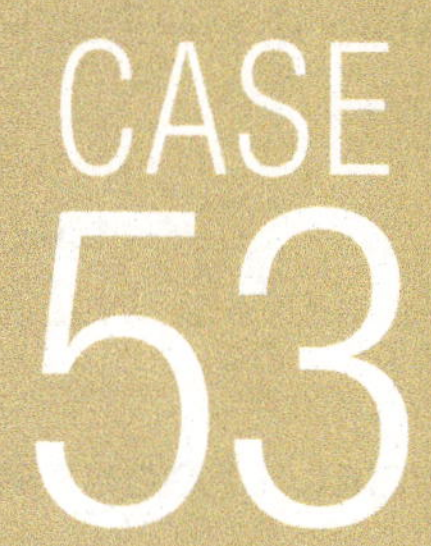

Chief Complaint

"Abdominal pain."

History of Present Illness

A 14-year-old boy, accompanied by his foster mother, presents to his PCP with abdominal pain that has been ongoing for 1 week. His foster mother is unable to pinpoint any more specific symptom description. He has no complaints of nausea, vomiting, diarrhea, or fever. He denies any aggravating or relieving factors. He does not eat spicy food, eats chocolate only occasionally, and does not skip meals. He drinks soda and orange juice occasionally. He does not drink coffee. He is unable to localize the pain. The consistency of his stool is soft. His appetite has decreased. He adds that he unable to sleep at night and is not sure why. His body language and the tone of his voice at this juncture seem as though he is scared and anxious about something. To put him at ease, the remainder of the history is taken with a chaperone and the foster mother is requested to step from the room. When asked if there is anything else that he would like to share, he opens up about what happened 2 months ago at a party. "It was a wild party, and everyone was hooking up." He really did not know anyone there but ended up "hooking up" with a girl he just met. He wanted to fit in at the party and is now worried that he may have caught something. He denies any penile discharge or dysuria.

Review of Systems

The patient's ROS is positive for anxiety, anorexia, insomnia, and abdominal pain. His ROS was negative for nausea, vomiting, diarrhea, constipation, fever, rash, and dysuria.

Relevant History

The patient has no chronic conditions and hospitalizations. His immunizations are up to date. He is in middle school and lives with a foster mother and three other foster children at home. His family history is unknown.

Allergies

No known drug allergies; no known food allergies.

Medications

None.

Physical Examination

- *Vitals:* T 37.0°C (98.7°F), P 100, R 20, BP 110/68, WT 50.8 kg (112 lb), HT 162.6 cm (64 in.), BMI 19.2.
- *General:* Alert and not in any distress.
- *Psychiatric:* Anxious.
- *Skin, Hair, and Nails:* Jaundice +. No signs of nail-biting or cuts on the wrist. No rash. No abnormal findings with hair or nails.
- *Eyes:* Red reflex intact. PERRL. No icterus.
- *Abdomen:* Nontender and soft on palpation. Not distended. BS are normal. No organomegaly or masses.

- *Genital/Rectal:* Normal penile and scrotal exam. No skin lesions noted. Rectal exam was deferred.
- *Neurologic:* A&O×3.

CLINICAL DISCUSSION QUESTIONS

1. What is the differential diagnosis?

2. What is the most likely diagnosis? Why?

3. Demonstrate your understanding about the pathophysiology of the most likely diagnosis.

4. Should tests/imaging studies be ordered? Which ones? Why? Think about tests/imaging beyond the primary care setting as well.

5. What are the next appropriate steps in management?

6. What are the prevalence, transmission, and screening of the diagnosis? Provide references for your response.

7. What are the pertinent ICD-10 and CPT (E/M) codes for this visit? Provide a short rationale.

8. What is the appropriate patient education topic for this case?

9. If not managed appropriately, what is/are the medical/legal concern(s) that may arise?

10. Think about interprofessional collaboration for this case. Provide a list of specialties or other disciplines and indicate what contribution these professionals might make to managing the patient.

BEDSIDE MANNER QUESTIONS

11. What would your communication style/approach be with this patient and his mother?

12. If the patient or his guardian is distressed by the diagnosis, what might offer support?

Answers available at courseconnect.springerpub.com.

CASE 54

SORE THROAT AND ABDOMINAL PAIN, ADOLESCENT MALE

Chief Complaint

"Sore throat and abdominal pain."

History of Present Illness

A 15-year-old boy presents to the clinic with his mother and brother following a 2-day history of throat and stomach pain. His mother reports that he has experienced temperatures of 38.5 to 39.1°C (101.3 to 102.4°F) for the past 2 days. She has given him acetaminophen tablets to help with the fever and throat pain. He states that his throat feels swollen and painful. He says he does not have any congestion or coughing. He denies vomiting or diarrhea but attests to vague pain in the upper areas of his abdomen that does not radiate. Additionally, he feels as though he cannot stay awake and has been napping in the mornings and afternoons. He has had to miss hockey practice for the past 2 days due to fever and illness and wants to know when he will be able to resume activity.

Review of Systems

The patient's ROS is positive for fever, sore throat, fatigue, and upper abdominal pain. His ROS is negative for vomiting, diarrhea, difficulty talking, coughing, rhinorrhea, sinus pressure, nasal congestion, nausea, heartburn, dyspepsia, rashes, weight loss, and lymphadenopathy.

Relevant History

The patient's medical history is significant for asthma that has resolved with age. He has seasonal allergies for which he takes levocetirizine 5 mg QD PRN. He does not consume alcohol or smoke. He reports no illicit drug usage. He states he is not sexually active and has had no recent kissing or sharing of utensils/cups. He is up to date on his vaccines, including Hib. His family history is significant for DM and heart disease. He is in the 10th grade, does well in school, and is a member of the hockey team which is in session during the present wintertime.

Allergies

No known drug allergies; no known food allergies.

Medications

Levocetirizine 5 mg QD PRN.

Physical Examination

- *Vitals:* T 39°C (102.2°F), P 92, R 16, BP 110/70 mmHG, HT 162.56 cm (64 in), WT 56.7 kg (125 lb), BMI 21.5.
- *General:* Well developed, well nourished, alert and cooperative, and appears to be in no acute distress.
- *Skin, Hair, and Nails:* No rashes. Skin is warm and dry without signs of jaundice. No abnormal findings with hair or nails, including the absence of discoloration, brittleness, or irregular growth patterns.
- *ENT/Mouth:* Oropharyngeal and tonsillar area with significant erythema, petechia, and white exudate; no stridor noted; no uvular deviation noted; patient is tolerating oral secretions; no tripod position noted. No changes in voice.

- *Neck:* Neck is soft, supple, with adequate ROM; no nuchal rigidity noted; tender, firm, rubbery BL adenopathy in the anterior and posterior cervical chain present. About 1.5 cm size.
- *Lungs:* CTA and percussion without rales, rhonchi, wheezing, or diminished breath sounds.
- *Heart:* Normal S1 and S2. RRR.
- *Abdomen:* Positive BS × 4 quadrants. Soft, nondistended. Remarkable tenderness to gentle palpation of the upper left quadrant. Mild tenderness to gentle palpation of the upper right quadrant. Presence of splenomegaly. No suprapubic, RLQ, or LLQ tenderness. Negative psoas sign, obturator sign, Rovsing sign; no tenderness at McBurney point.

Clinical Discussion Questions

1. What is the differential diagnosis?

2. What is the most likely diagnosis? Why?

3. Demonstrate your understanding about the pathophysiology of the most likely diagnosis.

4. Should tests/imaging studies be ordered? Which ones? Why? Think about tests/imaging beyond the primary care setting as well.

5. What are the next appropriate steps in management?

6. What are the testing recommendations, treatment options, and screening guidelines for this diagnosis? Provide references for your response.

7. What are the pertinent ICD-10 and CPT (E/M) codes for this visit? Provide a short rationale.

8. What is the appropriate patient education topic for this case?

9. If not managed appropriately, what is/are the medical/legal concern(s) that may arise?

10. Think about interprofessional collaboration for this case. Provide a list of specialties or other disciplines and indicate what contribution these professionals might make to managing the patient.

BEDSIDE MANNER QUESTION

11. What would your communication style/approach be with this patient and his mother?

____

____

____

____

Answers available at courseconnect.springerpub.com.

CASE 55

DOES NOT FOLLOW DIRECTIONS, PEDIATRIC MALE

Chief Complaint

"Child does not follow directions."

History of Present Illness

A mother brings her 8-year-old son to a PCP to evaluate his difficulty following directions. She states this has always been a problem at home and school. His teacher is concerned this year as he is not completing in-class assignments. In addition, he makes careless mistakes on his work, is easily distracted, and loses things. He interrupts the teacher frequently and fidgets in his seat. He gets along well with other children and seems to want to obey the teacher but has a hard time remembering what he is to do. He has not received any detentions or suspensions, and his mother states he is not a troublemaker at home or school.

Review of Systems

The patient's ROS is negative for palpitations, SOB, and chest pain; no chronic cough or wheeze; no snoring or difficulty sleeping; no pruritus, allergic rhinitis, or eczema; no abdominal pain, diarrhea, constipation, or vomiting. There is no history of anxiety, depression, or behavioral problems. No hospitalizations, chronic medical problems, or surgeries. The child sees a pediatric dentist every 6 months.

Relevant History

Tympanostomy tubes were inserted at 18 months and speech therapy for an expressive speech delay from 15 months until therapy ended at age 3. The boy was full-term; it was a normal pregnancy. There is no maternal alcohol, drug, or nicotine use, and the mother is G1P1. The child has no risk of exposure to lead. There is no family history of anxiety or depression. The boy's father struggled academically and was a "busy boy" in the classroom and at home. The family does not have a history of other mental illness or substance use or abuse or of cognitive delay or intellectual disability.

Allergies

No known drug allergies; no known food allergies.

Medications

None.

Physical Examination

- *Vitals:* T 37°C (98.6°F), P 72, R 15, BP 107/66, HT 129.50 cm (51 in.), WT 24.95 kg (55 lb), BMI 14.9.
- *General:* Well-developed, well-nourished cooperative child in no acute distress. No atypical facies noted.
- *Skin, Hair, and Nails:* No rashes or lesions noted.
- *Head:* Normocephalic and atraumatic.
- *Eyes:* PERRL; EOMI.
- *ENT/Mouth:* TMs pearly gray, mobile. Clear nasal discharge. Posterior oropharynx clear with small amount of postnasal drip. Tonsils 2+ and equal bilaterally.
- *Neck:* No cervical lymphadenopathy. No goiter noted.

- *Lungs:* CTA bilaterally; breath sounds equal.
- *Heart:* RRR; no murmur noted.
- *Abdomen:* Soft, nontender, and nondistended.
- *Genital/Rectal:* Sexual maturity rating stage 1; testicles descended bilaterally.
- *Neurologic:* CN II to XII grossly intact. Upper extremity and lower extremity strength 5/5 and equal bilaterally. Reflexes 2+ upper and lower extremities. Sensation normal upper and lower extremities. Gait is normal.

CLINICAL DISCUSSION QUESTIONS

1. What is the differential diagnosis?

2. What is the most likely diagnosis? Why?

3. Demonstrate your understanding about the pathophysiology of the most likely diagnosis.

4. Should tests/imaging studies be ordered? Which ones? Why? Think about tests/imaging beyond the primary care setting as well.

5. What are the next appropriate steps in management?

6. What are the diagnostic criteria and treatment options for this diagnosis? Provide references for your response.

7. What are the pertinent ICD-10 and CPT (E/M) codes for this visit? Provide a short rationale.

8. What is the appropriate patient education topic for this case?

9. If not managed appropriately, what is/are the medical/legal concern(s) that may arise?

10. Think about interprofessional collaboration for this case. Provide a list of specialties or other disciplines and indicate what contribution these professionals might make to managing the patient.

BEDSIDE MANNER QUESTIONS

11. What would your communication style/approach be with this patient and his mother?

12. If a patient and his mother are distressed by the diagnosis, what might offer support?

____

____

____

____

Answers available at courseconnect.springerpub.com.

CASE 56

CRUSTY, IRRITATED LEFT EYE, PEDIATRIC MALE

Chief Complaint

"Crusty, irritated left eye."

History of Present Illness

A mother brings her 5-year-old son to his PCP with a complaint of a 3-day history of a "crusty and irritated" OS. This morning, the mother noticed increased erythema and crusty white drainage to the lashes and inner canthus. No medications or other treatments were given. The mother is wondering if it is pinkeye because the day care center the child attends notified parents yesterday that a child was diagnosed with it. The mother is requesting medication for the child to start treatment along with asking if it is contagious and if she needs to take off from work to care for the child. She is concerned because she does not have the financial means to take time off work.

Review of Systems

The ROS is positive for OS erythema and pruritus with white crusty drainage. The ROS is negative for pain or change in visual acuity, photosensitivity, or recent trauma. The mother denies the child has had a fever or change in appetite and energy. There is no ear pain, nasal congestion, sore throat, headache, cough, SOB, rash, or muscle aches. The mother denies a recent viral URI or ear infection and reports no environmental or food allergies nor history of allergic rhinitis.

Relevant History

There is no significant medical history of concern. The child is generally healthy and was a normal birth. The patient takes no routine medications. There have been no surgeries or hospitalizations. The family history is unremarkable. It is a nonsmoking home. The child lives with his mother and older brother. He attends kindergarten and an after-school daycare program.

Allergies

No known drug allergies; no known food allergies.

Medications

None.

Physical Examination

- *Vitals:* T 37°C (98.6°F), P 92, R 20, BP 106/54, WT 9.07 kg (46 lb), HT 104.14 cm (41 in.), BMI 20.2.
- *General:* The patient is in no apparent distress except for rubbing his eyes. He is acting appropriate for his age, is clean and dressed well, and has a caring mother at his side.
- *Psychiatric:* Cooperative.
- *Skin, Hair, and Nails:* Rest of the exam with no abnormal finding.
- *Head:* Normocephalic.
- *Eyes:* Left conjunctiva erythema with lid swelling and a small amount of yellow purulent drainage to the lashes. Right conjunctiva is normal. There is no visual acuity deficit. No foreign body. PERRL. Red reflex intact bilaterally.
- *Snellen Test:* OD 20/20, OS 20/20, OU 20/20.

- *ENT/Mouth:* TMs present bilaterally with no ear drainage or tenderness to palpation. There is no preauricular lymphadenopathy. BL nares are without erythema, edema, or drainage. Oral mucosa is moist and normal. Normal dentation. Pharynx is normal.
- *Neck:* No cervical lymphadenopathy. FROM.
- *Lungs:* CTA bilaterally.
- *Heart:* RRR. No murmur.
- *Abdomen:* BS present. Abdomen soft with no tenderness to palpation.
- *Musculoskeletal:* Moves all extremities well with good strength.
- *Neurologic:* A&O×3.

Clinical Discussion Questions

1. What is the differential diagnosis?

2. What is the most likely diagnosis? Why?

3. Demonstrate your understanding about the pathophysiology of the most likely diagnosis.

4. Should tests/imaging studies be ordered? Which ones? Why? Think about tests/imaging beyond the primary care setting as well.

5. What are the next appropriate steps in management?

6. Review a recent and credible research article on making this diagnosis. Demonstrate your understanding of the treatment options and diagnostic criteria. Provide references.

7. What are the pertinent ICD-10 and CPT (E/M) codes for this visit? Provide a short rationale.

8. What is the appropriate patient education topic for this case?

9. If not managed appropriately, what is/are the medical/legal concern(s) that may arise?

10. Think about interprofessional collaboration for this case. Provide a list of specialties or other disciplines and indicate what contribution these professionals might make to managing the patient.

Bedside Manner Questions

11. What would your communication style/approach be with this patient and his mother?

12. If a patient and his mother are distressed by the diagnosis, what might offer support?

Answers available at courseconnect.springerpub.com.

CASE 57

CHEST PAIN WITH EXERTION, ADOLESCENT MALE

Chief Complaint

"Experiencing chest pain while running, especially during soccer games."

History of Present Illness

A 12-year-old male, an avid soccer player with no prior medical history, presents to the clinic with a concerning history of recurrent chest pain that has been manifesting for approximately 2 months. The episodes of chest pain are specifically triggered during physical exertion, notably after 20 to 30 minutes of playing soccer. The pain is described as a sharp, localized discomfort in the left anterior chest wall and/or the substernal area, which is the area of the chest overlying the heart. The intensity of the pain varies but has been significant enough to cause him to stop playing and take breaks during games.

The patient reports that the pain typically resolves upon cessation of physical activity. He has not noticed any progressive worsening or intensification of the symptoms over the last 2 months. There have been occasional episodes of excessive sweating associated with the painful episodes.

In addition to chest pain, the patient reports occasional episodes of lightheadedness that coincide with the pain. These episodes are transient but have raised concerns for the patient and his family. There have been no instances of syncope (fainting), palpitations, or SOB. The symptoms have not been associated with meals, emotional stress, or other specific triggers apart from physical exertion.

The patient has not taken any OTC medications for the symptoms and has no history of obesity, high cholesterol, HTN, DM, or mental health issues (anxiety/depression). There is no known family history of CVD or sudden cardiac death at a young age.

The patient sought initial advice from a school nurse who recommended further medical evaluation, given the recurrent nature of the symptoms and their association with physical activity. This prompted the current visit for a more comprehensive assessment and diagnosis, with a particular focus on evaluating for potential underlying CV conditions.

Review of Systems

The patient denies any history of palpitations, SOB, or syncope. He also denies any symptoms of fever, chills, or other constitutional symptoms. The patient has not noticed any recent significant weight gain or loss. There has been no presence of cyanosis. The patient has no history of wheezing or cough. The patient denies experiencing an irregular heartbeat. There have been no complaints of difficulty breathing when lying down. The patient reports no episodes of vomiting. There is no presence of lower extremity edema.

Relevant History

The patient's medical history is largely unremarkable, with no previous diagnoses of HTN, DM, or any other chronic conditions that could potentially be linked to CV issues. He has not undergone any surgical procedures. His immunizations are uptodate, including the standard pediatric vaccinations.

The family history is equally noncontributory, with no immediate family members having been diagnosed with early-onset CVDs, arrhythmias, or other heart conditions. There is no known history of sudden cardiac death or unexplained syncope in the family. Both parents are alive and well, with no chronic illnesses.

The patient's lifestyle is active, primarily centered around school and sports activities. He has been playing soccer for the past 4 years and has participated in other sports like swimming and basketball without any prior issues. He has no history of smoking, alcohol consumption, or substance abuse. His diet is described as balanced, without excessive intake of fast food, sugary beverages, or high-cholesterol foods.

Psychosocially, the patient is welladjusted, performing well in school, and maintaining healthy relationships with peers and family. He has not reported any significant stressors, either academically or socially, that could contribute to his symptoms.

Allergies

No known drug allergies; no known food allergies.

Medications

None.

Physical Examination

- *Vitals:* T 37°C (98.6°F), P 85, R 18, BP 120/75, WT 50 kg (110), HT 157.5 cm (62 in.), BMI 20.1.
- *General:* The patient appears to be a well-nourished, A&O 12-year-old male in no acute distress. He is cooperative and communicates clearly about his symptoms.
- *Cardiovascular:* Upon auscultation, a significant murmur is noted. The murmur is best heard at the left upper sternal border and is graded as 3/6 in intensity. It has a harsh quality and is holosystolic in timing. The first and second heart sounds (S1 and S2) are noted to be normal, with a regular rate and rhythm. No additional heart sounds, clicks, or gallop rhythms are detected. There are no signs of lifts, heaves, or thrills on the precordium. The PMI is not enlarged or displaced.

  Neck examination reveals no JVD. Peripheral pulses are checked and found to be symmetrical and strong in both upper and lower extremities, bilaterally. Capillary refill time is less than 2 seconds, and there is no evidence of lower extremity edema.

  The patient did the Valsalva technique, which made the murmur louder. When the patient stood up from squatting, the murmur became much louder.
- *Respiratory:* Lungs are CTA bilaterally, with no wheezing, crackles, or rhonchi noted. Respiratory effort is unlabored.
- *Musculoskeletal:* Muscle tone and strength are within normal limits. No deformities or limitations in joint movements are observed. The patient's posture is upright, and gait is normal.
- *Abdominal:* The abdomen is soft, nontender, and nondistended. No hepatosplenomegaly or masses are palpable. BS are normal in all quadrants.
- *Neurologic:* The patient is A&O×3 CN II to XII are intact. Sensory and motor functions are normal. Deep tendon reflexes are 2+ and symmetrical.
- *Skin:* No cyanosis, pallor, or jaundice is observed. Skin is warm and dry to the touch.

Clinical Discussion Questions

1. What is the differential diagnosis?

____

____

____

____

2. What is the most likely diagnosis? Why?

3. Demonstrate your understanding about the pathophysiology of the most likely diagnosis.

4. Should tests/imaging studies be ordered? Which ones? Why? Think about tests/imaging beyond the primary care setting as well.

5. What are the next appropriate steps in management?

6. What are the treatment options for this diagnosis? Provide references for your response.

7. What are the pertinent ICD-10 and CPT (E/M) codes for this visit? Provide a short rationale.

8. What is the appropriate patient education topic for this case?

9. If not managed appropriately, what is/are the medical/legal concern(s) that may arise?

10. Think about interprofessional collaboration for this case. Provide a list of specialties or other disciplines and indicate what contribution these professionals might make to managing the patient.

Bedside Manner Questions

11. What would your communication style/approach be with this family?

12. If a patient or his family is distressed by the diagnosis, what might offer support?

Answers available at courseconnect.springerpub.com.

CASE 58

DIFFICULTY RELATING TO OTHERS, PEDIATRIC MALE

Chief Complaint

"Difficulty relating to others."

History of Present Illness

A mother brings her 4-year-old son to their PCP to address his difficulties at home and school over the past 2 months. His preschool teacher requested a meeting last week and reported to the mother that her son seems to not pay attention during class. He stares off and often does not answer or make eye contact with her when she asks a question. The teacher also said he often stands up during class and walks around the room, disturbing his classmates. During group activities, he often gets upset with peers and repeats the phrase "doing it wrong" until he is allowed to finish the task alone. Despite all of this, he demonstrates mastery of the material. The mother explains that her son does not look her in the eyes often and that she often needs to say something to him a few times before he responds. He had been receiving early intervention speech therapy and OT since he was 15 months old. She states the interventions helped and were discontinued at age 2, but he continued some behaviors that have now worsened. He has never really been interested in playing with his siblings, but now he gets upset and cries if they try to play with him. The mother states he would spend hours playing with his toy cars if she let him, putting them in rows and then back in their containers. She has noticed he is picky about food. A speech therapist was able to get him to eat a few new foods, but now, on most days, he only wants chicken nuggets and mashed potatoes. Overall, his mother's main concern is his ability to continue in school and make some friends.

Review of Systems

The ROS is positive for changes in appetite and mood. All other symptoms are negative.

Relevant History

The child's medical history is significant for speech and fine motor delays diagnosed at 13 months. He received speech therapy and OT from age 15 months to 24 months. He was a full-term baby and the pregnancy was uncomplicated. All newborn screenings were normal. The child has had no significant illnesses and is up to date on immunizations.

The child lives with his parents and two siblings (ages 5 and 9). He sleeps 8 hours a night and often takes a 1-hour afternoon nap. He attends a half day of preschool in the morning. His mother works part-time in the morning while he is at school but is otherwise home with him. He sits in a booster seat in the car and wears a helmet when riding his bicycle. There are no firearms in the house or no secondhand smoke exposure. There is no significant family history.

Allergies

No known drug allergies; no known food allergies.

Medications

Daily multivitamin.

PHYSICAL EXAMINATION

- *Vitals:* T 37°C (98.6°F), P 82, R 18, BP 92/58, WT 18 kg (39.7 lb), HT 101.5 cm (39.75 in.), BMI 17.5.
- *General:* No acute distress but agitated during exam, sitting quietly next to mother playing with toy car.
- *Psychiatric:* Complies with exam but disinterested, answers questions with short responses, little eye contact with mother or provider, spinning/examining wheels of toy car repetitively throughout exam.
- *Skin, Hair, and Nails:* Skin warm and dry; no rashes, lesions, bruising, or discoloration.
- *Head:* Normocephalic and atraumatic.
- *Eyes:* PERRLA; EOMI.
- *ENT/Mouth:* Ear canal clear, TMs visible bilaterally without erythema or effusion, nares patent, turbinates pink and moist, good oral hygiene, oropharynx mucosa pink and moist.
- *Neck:* No masses, no lymphadenopathy.
- *Lungs:* CTA bilaterally.
- *Heart:* RRR, no murmurs.
- *Abdomen:* BS active, soft, nontender, nondistended.
- *Musculoskeletal:* Strength 5/5 upper and lower extremities.
- *Neurologic:* CN II to XII grossly intact, good muscle tone.

CLINICAL DISCUSSION QUESTIONS

1. What is the differential diagnosis?

2. What is the most likely diagnosis? Why?

3. Demonstrate your understanding about the pathophysiology of the most likely diagnosis.

4. Should tests/imaging studies be ordered? Which ones? Why? Think about tests/imaging beyond the primary care setting as well.

5. What are the next appropriate steps in management?

6. According to the most recent research, what are the key factors in making the diagnosis and the prevalence of the diagnosis? Provide references for your response.

7. What are the pertinent ICD-10 and CPT (E/M) codes for this visit? Provide a short rationale.

8. What is the appropriate patient education topic for this case?

9. If not managed appropriately, what is/are the medical/legal concern(s) that may arise?

10. Think about interprofessional collaboration for this case. Provide a list of specialties or other disciplines and indicate what contribution these professionals might make to managing the patient.

Bedside Manner Questions

11. What would your communication style/approach be with this patient's mother?

12. If a patient's mother is distressed by the diagnosis, what might offer support?

Answers available at courseconnect.springerpub.com.

FEVER AND LUMP ON NECK, ADOLESCENT MALE

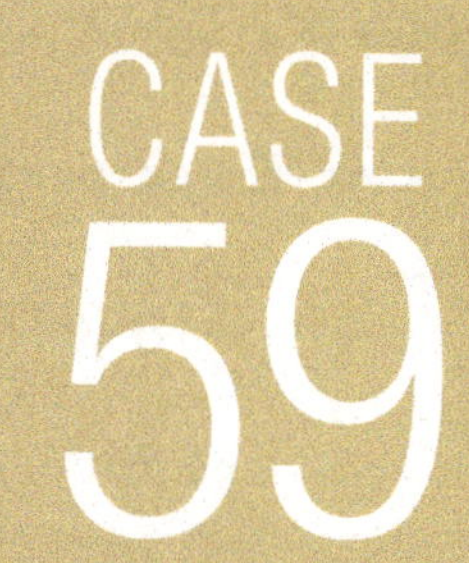

Chief Complaint

"Fever and lump on neck."

History of Present Illness

A 13-year-old boy presents to an urban FQHC reporting a lump on the left side of his neck, just below his ear, that has been there for 6 days. The patient speaks English, but his mother, who brings him to the clinic, only speaks Spanish. A trained medical Spanish interpreter attends the patient interview. The patient noticed a small bump on his neck one night 6 days ago. The following day, the lump became larger and the patient developed a fever. The fever was subjective, meaning the family did not take his temperature, but he felt feverish and was warm to the touch. On the evening of onset, he had a transient rash, which the mother describes as "hives." He complained of a sore throat the previous week but denies a sore throat currently. He does report slight dysphagia and mild headache.

He was seen 4 days earlier by another provider in the same clinic and started on amoxicillin for presumed bacterial lymphadenitis. At that time, he was febrile: 100.8°F (38.2°C). The mass is described as a 2.5- to 3-cm submandibular gland enlargement, which is firm and tender to palpation. A CBC was normal, and group A strep, mumps, and EBV testing were negative. Since that time, the patient thinks the lump has grown in size. His headache is somewhat improved, but he continues to be febrile.

Review of Systems

The patient's ROS is positive for a slight cough. His ROS is negative for abdominal pain, nausea, vomiting, or diarrhea. There is no eye discharge, pain, or irritation. There are no ear symptoms or nasal symptoms. There are no current skin symptoms, and the skin overlying the lump is not red or draining.

Relevant History

The patient's history is significant for atopic dermatitis, which has not been active within the past 6 months. There are no other known medical conditions. The patient has never been hospitalized, nor has he ever had surgery. Immunizations are up to date.

The patient lives with his parents, who are married, and his two siblings. The family is Spanish-speaking, but the patient himself speaks fluent English. The family emigrated from El Salvador when the patient was a small child. The patient is uninsured, and the family is on a sliding fee scale at the FQHC. The patient has two pet kittens who sleep in his bedroom. There are no other pets and no environmental tobacco smoke exposure. There has been no recent travel. The family lives in a home built within the past 30 years and has city water.

Allergies

No known drug allergies. No known food allergies.

Medications

- Amoxicillin 250 mg, PO TID for the past 4 days. Last dose was about 6 hours ago.
- Acetaminophen 325 mg, two tablets PO Q8h. Last dose was about 6 hours ago.

Physical Examination

- *Vitals:* T 37.2°C (99.0°F); P 77; R 16; BP 103/60; HT 157.5 cm (62 in.), 30th percentile; WT 45 kg. (99 lb), 31st percentile; BMI 18.2, 38th percentile.
- *General:* A&O, in no acute distress, with obvious swelling on the left jaw line at the angle of the mandible.
- *Psychiatric:* Appropriate interaction for age. Affect is full and mood is regular.
- *Skin, Hair, and Nails:* Scattered superficial abrasions noted on BL UEs, which the patient states are from his kittens and do not hurt. No abnormal findings with hair or nails.
- *Eyes:* Sclerae clear.
- *ENT/Mouth:* Ear canals are patent, and TMs are clear. Mouth mucosa is pink and moist without erythema, inflammation, or exudate.
- *Neck:* Some limit to ROM secondary to a firm, but not hard, mobile 3×4-cm left-sided submandibular mass. The mass is tender to palpation without significant overlying induration or erythema but is slightly warm to the touch. There is no other anterior, occipital, or supraclavicular lymphadenopathy appreciated.
- *Lungs:* CTA bilaterally.
- *Heart:* RRR without murmurs, rubs, or gallops.
- *Abdomen:* Soft, nontender, nondistended, with no organomegaly.
- *Genital/Rectal:* Deferred.
- *Neurologic:* No focal deficits. CN II to XII are normal.

Clinical Discussion Questions

1. What is the differential diagnosis?

2. What is the most likely diagnosis? Why?

3. Demonstrate your understanding about the pathophysiology of the most likely diagnosis.

4. Should tests/imaging studies be ordered? Which ones? Why? Think about tests/imaging beyond the primary care setting as well.

5. What are the next appropriate steps in management?

6. What is the treatment approach for this diagnosis? Provide references for your response.

7. What are the pertinent ICD-10 and CPT (E/M) codes for this visit? Provide a short rationale.

8. What is the appropriate patient education topic for this case?

9. If not managed appropriately, what is/are the medical/legal concern(s) that may arise?

10. Think about interprofessional collaboration for this case. Provide a list of specialties or other disciplines and indicate what contribution these professionals might make to managing the patient.

BEDSIDE MANNER QUESTION

11. What would your communication style/approach be with this parent and patient?

Answers available at courseconnect.springerpub.com.

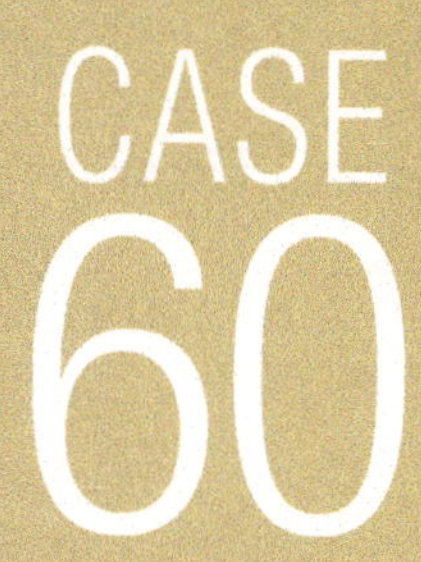

CASE 60

RECURRENT VOMITING, PEDIATRIC FEMALE

Chief Complaint

"Recurrent vomiting."

History of Present Illness

A mother presents with her 3-year-old daughter for an evaluation of recurrent vomiting. At the time of her first office visit, the patient had a 3- to 4-day history of one or two episodes of vomiting daily. There were no associated symptoms, and she had no ill contacts. A physical examination of the skin, ears, throat, neck, thorax, and abdomen showed no abnormalities. A diagnosis of viral syndrome was made, and she was sent home with dietary modifications.

Despite slight improvement with dietary modifications, the child continued to have sporadic episodes of vomiting one to three times daily. She remained afebrile and, apart from a decreased appetite, had no new symptoms. Because of the persistent vomiting, she was seen in the clinic again 2 days later by a different provider. Her weight had decreased from 31 lb to 29.5 lb, but she showed no signs of dehydration and her abdominal examination showed no abnormalities. At this visit, the provider discussed with the mother that although the time course of her vomiting was prolonged for a viral illness, she appeared well hydrated and had no concerning findings on abdominal examination. The mother was advised to encourage clear liquids and to offer small amounts of solids as tolerated. A follow-up appointment was scheduled for 3 days later.

The day before the scheduled follow-up appointment, the mother called the office concerned about the child's continued vomiting. The call was transferred to the provider who had seen her most recently, and her mother told the PCP, "I just know something is wrong. I'm afraid we're going to lose her." Because of this concern, the PCP recommended that the child be evaluated that same morning. Further history revealed that since her last visit, she had continued to have sporadic episodes of emesis, and when asked what concerned her most, her mother explained that this illness just seemed different from any she had experienced before. The vomiting seems to occur without warning, and she "just isn't acting herself."

Review of Systems

The patient's ROS is positive for weight loss, decreased appetite, and decreased activity. Her ROS is negative for fever, headache, nausea, abdominal pain, hematemesis, bilious emesis, cramping, diarrhea, or hematochezia.

Relevant History

The patient was diagnosed with GERD, diagnosed at age 6 months; she was treated with frequent, smaller feedings and thickening formula. The GERD resolved by 15 months of age.

Allergies

No known drug allergies; no known food allergies.

Medications

None.

PHYSICAL EXAMINATION

- *Vitals:* T 37°C (98.4°F), P 94, R 22, BP 90/50, HT 86 cm (34 in.), WT 12.7 kg (28 lb), BMI 17.0.
- *General:* Alert, sitting comfortably on mother's lap.
- *Skin, Hair, and Nails:* No rash or skin lesions, normal skin turgor.
- *Eyes:* No conjunctival injection or scleral icterus, PERRL.
- *ENT/Mouth:* Oropharynx without lesions, mucosa moist.
- *Neck:* FROM, nontender, no lymphadenopathy.
- *Lungs:* CTA bilaterally.
- *Heart:* RRR, S1 and S2 normal intensity, no murmur or extra heart sounds.
- *Abdomen:* Nondistended; normal quality and frequency of BS; soft, nontender to deep palpation; no mass or hepatosplenomegaly.
- *Neurologic:* CN II to XII intact bilaterally, normal strength upper and lower extremity, gait wide based and unsteady.

CLINICAL DISCUSSION QUESTIONS

1. What is the differential diagnosis?

____

____

____

____

2. What is the most likely diagnosis? Why?

____

____

____

____

3. Demonstrate your understanding about the pathophysiology of the most likely diagnosis.

____

____

____

____

4. Should tests/imaging studies be ordered? Which ones? Why? Think about tests/imaging beyond the primary care setting as well.

____

____

____

____

5. What are the next appropriate steps in management?

6. Review a credible research article/s about this diagnosis. Demonstrate your understanding of the prevalence, treatment options, and risks. Provide your reference(s).

7. What are the pertinent ICD-10 and CPT (E/M) codes for this visit? Provide a short rationale.

8. What is the appropriate patient education topic for this case?

9. If not managed appropriately, what is/are the medical/legal concern(s) that may arise?

10. Think about interprofessional collaboration for this case. Provide a list of specialties or other disciplines and indicate what contribution these professionals might make to managing the patient.

BEDSIDE MANNER QUESTIONS

11. What would your communication style/approach be with this parent?

12. If a parent and child are distressed by the diagnosis, what might offer support?

Answers available at courseconnect.springerpub.com.

CASE 61

NAUSEA, VOMITING, AND HEADACHE, ADOLESCENT MALE

Chief Complaint

"Nausea, vomiting, and headache."

History of Present Illness

A mother brings her 13-year-old son to his PCP for evaluation. He has a 1-day history of nausea, vomiting, and headache with photosensitivity. He is in the 8th grade, doing well in school, and active in community sports. During a football game yesterday, the front of his head connected with another player's shoulder pads; his head whipped back; he lost his balance; and he fell to the ground, hitting the back of his head. His mother helps recount the accident, as the patient does not remember all the details. No loss of consciousness was noted. After a brief rest on the sidelines, he continued minimal play. The team went for pizza after the game; during dinner, he complained of a headache. Upon arriving at home, he had two to three episodes of nausea/vomiting. The headache continued with photosensitivity. Today, he has continued nausea, with no further vomiting; headache is still present, and he states, "My balance is a bit off."

Review of Systems

The patient's ROS is positive for nausea, vomiting, headache, mild visual changes, and mild balance disturbances. His ROS is negative for sleep difficulty or excessive sleep; difficulty concentrating; irritability; or sadness, numbness, or tingling.

Relevant History

The boy was born via Cesarean section at term, 8 lb, 19.5 in. There was a history of newborn GERD, which has resolved. He was the parents' first child. He lives with parents and siblings in a single-family home with no family history of smoking. His family medical history is negative, except for the mom with thyroid removal surgery in 2010 for a nodular noncancerous thyroid.

Allergies

No known drug allergies; no known food allergies.

Medications

None.

Physical Examination

- *Vitals:* T 37°C (98.7°F), P 98, BP 102/54, WT 59.3 kg (130.8 lb), HT 157.5 cm (62 in.), BMI 23.9.
- *General:* Alert and active in mild acute distress. Appears fatigued.
- *Psychiatric:* Affect is normal and appropriate.
- *Head:* Head is normocephalic.
- *Eyes:* PERRL, red reflex present bilaterally, EOM full, positive nystagmus.
- *ENT/Mouth:* TMs pearly gray with visible cone of light and landmarks. Mucosa is pink and moist. Normal speech and tone. Uvula midline.
- *Lungs:* Respirations even and unlabored, clear bilaterally.

- *Heart:* Normal S1 and S2 without rubs, murmurs, or gallops.
- *Musculoskeletal:* Motor 5/5 proximal and distal upper and lower extremities, including shoulders. DTRs 2+ and symmetrical of knees, Achilles, brachioradialis, and biceps tendons. Gait normal, balance distorted with standing on one foot and heal toe walking, has pronator drift.
- *Neurologic:* CN II to XII grossly intact. Sensory grossly intact to light touch symmetrically.

Clinical Discussion Questions

1. What is the differential diagnosis?

2. What is the most likely diagnosis? Why?

3. Demonstrate your understanding about the pathophysiology of the most likely diagnosis.

4. Should tests/imaging studies be ordered? Which ones? Why? Think about tests/imaging beyond the primary care setting as well.

5. What are the next appropriate steps in management?

6. What are the prevalence, complications, and current guidelines post diagnosis? Provide references for your response.

7. What are the pertinent ICD-10 and CPT (E/M) codes for this visit? Provide a short rationale.

8. What is the appropriate patient education topic for this case?

9. If not managed appropriately, what is/are the medical/legal concern(s) that may arise?

10. Think about interprofessional collaboration for this case. Provide a list of specialties or other disciplines and indicate what contribution these professionals might make to managing the patient.

BEDSIDE MANNER QUESTIONS

11. What would your communication style/approach be with this patient and his mother?

12. If the patient and his mother are distressed by the diagnosis, what might offer support?

____

____

____

____

Answers available at courseconnect.springerpub.com.

CASE 62

FREQUENT DIARRHEA, ADOLESCENT FEMALE

Chief Complaint

"Frequent diarrhea."

History of Present Illness

A 16-year-old young woman presents to her family PCP with her mother. The patient began having GI symptoms 2 years ago, following a camping trip with her family. At that time, both the patient and her older brother developed acute nausea, vomiting, abdominal pain, and diarrhea. No other family members were affected. The parents thought the children had a virus or food poisoning and treated them conservatively with oral fluid replacement and acetaminophen for low-grade fever. The brother's symptoms resolved quickly over the next 2 to 3 days; the patient's symptoms slowly improved over 1 week. However, since then, she has had recurrent episodes of lower abdominal cramping and pain, combined with loose to watery, nonbloody stools. At times, she will have a sense of fecal urgency and tenesmus associated with the diarrhea. She also frequently feels bloated. Her symptoms have occurred at least 1 day per week for the past 6 months. The patient also has occasional headaches that respond well to treatment with acetaminophen. Her appetite and weight have remained stable, and no other symptoms have developed.

The family's PCP first saw her a few weeks after the initial illness because of recurring symptoms and she has been seen in follow-up 2 to 3 times over the past year. During this time, several studies have been done: stool studies (ova and parasites, fecal leukocytes, routine stool cultures, and tests for *Giardia lamblia*), which were normal, and blood work (CBC, CMP, and CRP), which was normal. When her symptoms persisted, tests for celiac disease (serum TTG antibody and serum IgA) were done and were negative. The mother states they have avoided gluten and dairy products without long-term improvement. The only medication used is loperamide PRN. The use of loperamide has resulted in some improvement in the diarrhea, but the bloating and lower abdominal pain and cramps persist.

Review of Systems

The ROS was positive for the symptoms related in the HPI: abdominal pain, bloating, and diarrhea. The ROS was negative for fever, chills, vomiting, weight loss, urinary symptoms, and fatigue.

Relevant History

The patient has had no major illnesses, injuries, surgeries, or hospitalizations. Menstrual history: menarche at age 12. First day of LMP 14 days ago. Menses are regular, occurring every 28 to 30 days. Flow is moderate, lasting 5 to 7 days. She denies dysmenorrhea. She is not sexually active. There is no family history of cancer or IBD.

Allergies

No known drug allergies; no known food allergies.

Medications

Acetaminophen 500 mg PRN for fever and headaches.

PHYSICAL EXAMINATION

- *Vitals:* T 37°C (98.6°F), P 76, R 14, BP 114/72, HT 165 cm (65 in.), WT 53.5 kg (118 lb), BMI 19.6.
- *General:* Well-developed and nourished 16-year-old female patient in no acute distress.
- *Psychiatric:* Appears mildly anxious.
- *Skin, Hair, and Nails:* Skin warm and dry, no rashes or bleeding tendency.
- *ENT/Mouth:* Ears: TMs appear pearly; gray with no fluid noted. Oral mucosa is moist and dentition is in good repair with no caries or erosions.
- *Neck:* Supple with no adenopathy or thyroid enlargement.
- *Lungs:* CTA bilaterally.
- *Heart:* RRR, without murmur, gallop, or rub.
- *Abdomen:* Soft with no masses, organomegaly, or tenderness. Active BS heard in all quadrants.
- *Genital/Rectal:* Deferred.
- *Lymphatics:* No axillary or inguinal lymphadenopathy.
- *Neurologic:* A&O×3, CN II to XII grossly intact.

CLINICAL DISCUSSION QUESTIONS

1. What is the differential diagnosis?

____

____

____

____

2. What is the most likely diagnosis? Why?

____

____

____

____

3. Demonstrate your understanding about the pathophysiology of the most likely diagnosis.

____

____

____

____

4. Should tests/imaging studies be ordered? Which ones? Why? Think about tests/imaging beyond the primary care setting as well.

____

____

____

____

5. What are the next appropriate steps in management?

6. What are the diagnostic criteria and underlying conditions associated with the diagnosis? Include the name of the references.

7. What are the pertinent ICD-10 and CPT (E/M) codes for this visit? Provide a short rationale.

8. What is the appropriate patient education topic for this case?

9. If not managed appropriately, what is/are the medical/legal concern(s) that may arise?

10. Think about interprofessional collaboration for this case. Provide a list of specialties or other disciplines and indicate what contribution these professionals might make to managing the patient.

BEDSIDE MANNER QUESTIONS

11. What would your communication style/approach be with this patient and her mother?

12. If a patient and her mother are distressed by the diagnosis, what might offer support?

Answers available at courseconnect.springerpub.com.

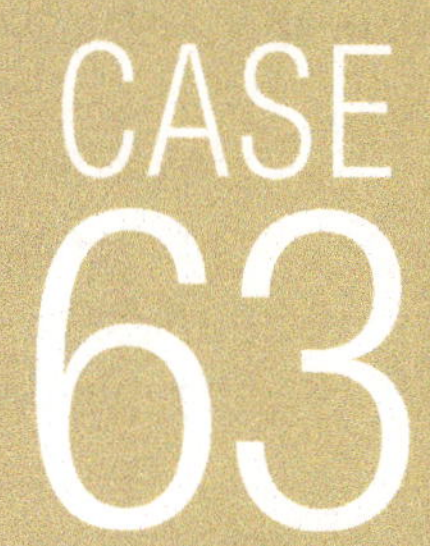

CASE 63

REPETITIVE BRUISING ON LEGS, PEDIATRIC FEMALE

Chief Complaint

"Repetitive bruising on legs."

History of Present Illness

A mother and her 16-month-old daughter present to their pediatric office with a 2-week history of bruising. The mother says 2 weeks ago, she started noticing bruises of different sizes primarily on the child's legs and thighs. After some bruises faded, new ones appeared. They start as purple spots and then change to brown before shrinking and disappearing. The child is walking now and stumbles but no more so than any toddler. She is active and energetic without any recent trauma/accidents. She has been seen regularly in the clinic for all her routine well-child checks, and bruising was not noted at the last 15-month well-child check, when she received immunizations. The mother mentions that the child had a cold about 3 weeks ago, but the low-grade fever and sniffles resolved in a few days. Currently, her daughter has no other symptoms. She demonstrates normal growth, normal development, and a healthy diet.

Review of Systems

The child's ROS is positive for bruises on BLE, recent viral illness 3 weeks ago, and routine vaccines 1 month ago. Her ROS is negative for fever; fatigue; nosebleeds; gingival bleeding; hematuria; hematochezia; change in appetite, energy, voids, and stools; and new medications.

Relevant History

The child has no previously recorded or active medical problems. She lives at home with her parents and older sibling and attends day care 3 days a week. Family history is negative for cancer, bleeding disorders, and autoimmune disorders.

Allergies

No known drug allergies; no known food allergies.

Medications

None.

Physical Examination

- *Vitals:* T 36.9°C (98.4°F); P 116; R 26; BP 100/60; WT 10.6 kg (23 lb, 6 oz.), 75th percentile; HT 80 cm (31.5 in.), 75th percentile; HC 46.2 cm (18.1 in.).
- *General:* Well appearing, interactive and playful, walking around the exam room, non-concerning interaction between parent and child.
- *Skin, Hair, and Nails:* No excessive pallor, 10 to 12 purple–brown macules with irregular borders of varying sizes from 0.5 to 2 cm in diameter on BL legs and thighs, nontender, non-blanching; also with 5 to 6 nonblanching, pinpoint, brightly erythematous macules on the forehead and left cheek.
- *ENT/Mouth:* Normal nasal turbinates with pink mucosa, no evidence of bleeding. Moist mucous membranes with no evidence of gingival bleeding, no thrush, normal pharynx.

- *Neck:* No cervical lymphadenopathy.
- *Axilla:* No axillary lymphadenopathy.
- *Abdomen:* Soft, nontender, nondistended, no hepatomegaly, no splenomegaly, no inguinal lymphadenopathy.

CLINICAL DISCUSSION QUESTIONS

1. What is the differential diagnosis?

2. What is the most likely diagnosis? Why?

3. Demonstrate your understanding about the pathophysiology of the most likely diagnosis.

4. Should tests/imaging studies be ordered? Which ones? Why? Think about tests/imaging beyond the primary care setting as well.

5. What are the next appropriate steps in management?

6. What are the causes and prognosis of the diagnosis? Provide references for your responses.

7. What are the pertinent ICD-10 and CPT (E/M) codes for this visit? Provide a short rationale.

8. What is the appropriate parent education topic for this case?

9. If not managed appropriately, what is/are the medical/legal concern(s) that may arise?

10. Think about interprofessional collaboration for this case. Provide a list of specialties or other disciplines and indicate what contribution these professionals might make to managing the patient.

BEDSIDE MANNER QUESTIONS

11. What would your communication style/approach be with this parent?

12. If a patient's mother is distressed by the diagnosis, what might offer support?

____

____

____

____

Answers available at courseconnect.springerpub.com.

CASE 64

ANXIETY ATTACKS AND NIGHTMARES, PEDIATRIC FEMALE

Chief Complaint

"Anxiety attacks, nightmares, flashbacks, and symptoms of hyperactivity and attention deficit."

History of Present Illness

A 7-year-old girl, accompanied by her mother, reports a complex array of symptoms progressively worsening over the last 2 years, closely following exposure to a traumatic event involving domestic violence between her parents. In the aftermath, she has been experiencing recurrent anxiety attacks, manifesting as palpitations, excessive sweating, and trembling, with these episodes occurring three to four times weekly. These anxiety attacks are frequently triggered by reminders of the domestic violence incident, leading to vivid flashbacks, which are experienced separately from her nightmares that disrupt her sleep approximately 5 nights a week.

In addition to her anxiety symptoms, she exhibits significant hyperactivity and attention deficits. She struggles to stay seated and maintain focus on tasks both in school and at home. It is uncertain whether these attention deficit symptoms were present before the traumatic event or are a secondary response to her anxiety. Social withdrawal is also notable, with the girl avoiding activities and interactions she once enjoyed. Episodes of impulsive physical aggression, particularly toward her mother, have been observed.

Review of Systems

The child presents with no significant constitutional, CV, respiratory, GI, musculoskeletal, or endocrine symptoms. Neurologically, there are no seizures, headaches, dizziness, or loss of consciousness reported. However, the patient endorses recurrent anxiety attacks with palpitations, excessive sweating, trembling, vivid flashbacks, nightmares disrupting sleep, and episodes of physical aggression. Additionally, there is a noted inability to stay seated, frequent daydreaming, and a lack of attention to detail. The patient also shows withdrawal from activities and social isolation. Notably, the child experiences significant sleep disturbances, with nightmares occurring approximately 5 nights a week. No changes in eating habits, substance use or exposures, or specific obsessive-compulsive behaviors are reported. There are also no reports of dysuria, hematuria, or skin changes.

Relevant History

The patient was born full-term via vaginal delivery with no complications during pregnancy or birth. Her developmental milestones were achieved within normal limits, and she had no significant medical history until the age of 5. At that time, she was exposed to a traumatic event involving domestic violence between her parents. This event led to her mother separating from her father, and they since have been living in a different, safer environment.

The patient's family history is significant for mental health disorders; her maternal grandmother was diagnosed with GAD, and her paternal uncle has a history of substance abuse. There are no known cases of ADHD in the family, but her older brother has been diagnosed with mild depression.

She has been attending regular school but has faced academic challenges since the onset of her symptoms. Her grades have declined, and she has been receiving additional support from the school's special education department. She has also been involved in IEPs to address her academic and behavioral issues.

Allergies

No known drug allergies; no known food allergies.

Medications

Children's daily multivitamin.

Physical Examination

- *Vitals:* T 36.8°C (98.2°F), P 90, R 18, BP 110/70 mmHg, HT 123 cm (48.4 in), WT 23 kg (50.7 lb), BMI 15.2.
- *General:* Appears anxious, frequently shifting in her seat, but cooperative and responsive to questions.
- *Psychiatric:* Displays signs of hyperactivity and restlessness. Eye contact is intermittent. Speech is rapid but coherent.
- *Skin, Hair, and Nails:* Skin appears normal, no rashes or lesions. Hair and nails are well groomed.
- *Head:* Normal cephalic, atraumatic. No signs of injury.
- *Lungs:* CTA bilaterally, no wheezing or crackles.
- *Heart:* RRR, no murmurs, or gallops. Pulses 2+ in all extremities.
- *Abdomen:* Soft, nontender, no masses or hepatosplenomegaly.
- *Neurologic:* A&O×3 Alert and oriented to person, place, and time. CN II to XII intact. DTRs 2+ and symmetric.

Clinical Discussion Questions

1. What is the differential diagnosis?

2. What is the most likely diagnosis? Why?

3. Demonstrate your understanding about the pathophysiology of the most likely diagnosis.

4. Should tests/imaging studies be ordered? Which ones? Why? Think about tests/imaging beyond the primary care setting as well.

5. What are the next appropriate steps in management?

6. Review recent and credible research article(s) on this diagnosis. Demonstrate your understanding about the treatment approach and pharmacology options. Provide references for your response(s).

7. What are the pertinent ICD-10 and CPT (E/M) codes for this visit? Provide a short rationale.

8. What is the appropriate patient education topic for this case?

9. If not managed appropriately, what is/are the medical/legal concern(s) that may arise?

10. Think about interprofessional collaboration for this case. Provide a list of specialties or other disciplines and indicate what contribution these professionals might make to managing the patient.

Bedside Manner Question

11. What would your communication style/approach be with this patient and her mother?

Answers available at courseconnect.springerpub.com.

WIDESPREAD PAINFUL RASH, PEDIATRIC FEMALE

CASE 65

Chief Complaint

"Widespread painful rash."

History of Present Illness

A mother and her 9-year-old daughter present to a pediatric clinic for a second opinion regarding the daughter's symptoms of fever, sore throat, and a painful rash. She had been seen 3 days earlier by her regular PCP, who diagnosed a viral infection. Her parents were concerned and sought a second opinion because she had a persistent high fever and her rash had worsened. The rash had extended to her extremities, had multiple areas of blistering, and continued to be painful. Within the past 24 hours, she developed sores on her lips and purulent discharge from both eyes. She is currently on day 9 of antibiotic treatment for uncomplicated cystitis.

Ten days prior to this visit, she had seen her regular PCP for evaluation of dysuria. She had no fever at that time. She was diagnosed with cystitis and prescribed a course of sulfamethoxazole-trimethoprim. The dysuria resolved within 24 hours and did not recur. Five days after starting the antibiotic, she developed a fever up to 40°C (104°F), generalized malaise, a mild sore throat, and skin pain. On day 6 of antibiotic treatment, she developed a rash on her face and trunk and was seen again by her PCP. Her parents stated that the rash was deep red and consisted of irregular blotchy areas with one or two small blisters. Her parents were told that her symptoms were most likely due to a viral infection because she was already taking an antibiotic.

They were advised to continue the antibiotic as prescribed and to give acetaminophen PRN for fever. No follow-up was scheduled.

Review of Systems

The patient's ROS is positive for generalized weakness, decreased appetite, eye pain, and photophobia. Her ROS is negative for headache, neck pain, vomiting, diarrhea, or abdominal pain.

Relevant History

The patient's history is significant for several episodes of OM, one previous episode of cystitis about 2 years earlier, and two episodes of streptococcal pharyngitis since starting kindergarten. There is no history of chronic illness. Her immunizations are up to date for her age.

Allergies

No known drug allergies; no known food allergies.

Medications

- Sulfamethoxazole-trimethoprim 400 mg/80 mg PO BID.
- Acetaminophen 325 mg PO QID PRN for pain.

PHYSICAL EXAMINATION

- *Vitals:* T 39.6°C (103.3°F), P 96, R 18, BP 92/56 mmHg, HT 127 cm (50 in.), WT 28.2 kg (62 lb), BMI 17.4.
- *General:* Ill appearing, in moderate discomfort.
- *Skin, Hair, and Nails:* Face, trunk, and extremities with extensive erythematous and dark purple irregularly shaped macules with overlying vesicles of varying sizes (up to approximately 3 to 4 cm in diameter) and areas of deep skin erosion covering a small percentage of total skin surface; skin tender to light touch. No abnormal findings with hair or nails.
- *Head:* No scalp lesions.
- *Eyes:* Moderate conjunctival injection with small amount of purulent discharge bilaterally.
- *ENT/Mouth:* TMs translucent with normal mobility, oropharynx with mild erythema, lips erythematous with several areas of erosion and crusting.
- *Neck:* FROM without discomfort; no resistance to flexion; no lymphadenopathy.
- *Lungs:* CTA bilaterally.
- *Heart:* RRR, S1 and S2 normal intensity, no murmurs or extra heart sounds.
- *Abdomen:* Soft, nontender; no mass or hepatosplenomegaly.
- *Genital/Rectal:* No lesions of external genitalia.
- *Musculoskeletal:* No joint swelling, FROM.
- *Neurologic:* Responds appropriately to questions; CNs intact; strength and sensation not assessed due to skin lesions and tenderness; walks but appears to be in pain with movement.

CLINICAL DISCUSSION QUESTIONS

1. What is the differential diagnosis?

____

____

____

____

2. What is the most likely diagnosis? Why?

____

____

____

____

3. Demonstrate your understanding about the pathophysiology of the most likely diagnosis.

____

____

____

____

4. Should tests/imaging studies be ordered? Which ones? Why? Think about tests/imaging beyond the primary care setting as well.

5. What are the next appropriate steps in management?

6. What are the causes, risk factors, and treatment for this diagnosis? Provide references for your responses.

7. What are the pertinent ICD-10 and CPT (E/M) codes for this visit? Provide a short rationale.

8. What is appropriate patient education topic for this case?

9. If not managed appropriately, what is/are the medical/legal concern(s) that may arise?

10. Think about interprofessional collaboration for this case. Provide a list of specialties or other disciplines and indicate what contribution these professionals might make to managing the patient.

BEDSIDE MANNER QUESTIONS

11. What would your communication style/approach be with this mother and patient?

12. If a patient and her mother are distressed by the diagnosis, what might offer support?

Answers available at courseconnect.springerpub.com.

CASE 66

BAD COUGH AND FEVER, ADOLESCENT FEMALE

Chief Complaint

"Bad cough and fever."

History of Present Illness

A 14-year-old girl is brought to her PCP's office in the month of December by her mother. The patient has had a cough for 5 days and fever for 2 days with a maximum temperature at home of 39.5°C (103.1°F), tympanic, taken last night. Her symptoms began with nasal congestion and sore throat 5 days ago, along with a mild cough that has progressed over the last 48 hours to become productive and more severe and with two episodes of post-tussive emesis. The patient occasionally is short of breath and complains of chills.

Review of Systems

The patient's ROS is positive for malaise; intermittent headache; nasal congestion, rhinorrhea, sore throat, cough, and occasional dyspnea; post-tussive emesis; fever; chill; and chest pain with cough. The ROS is negative for vision or hearing disturbances, otalgia, neck pain or stiffness, wheezing, nausea, diarrhea, constipation, abdominal pain, rash, urinary symptoms, or arthralgia.

Relevant History

The patient's medical history is unremarkable and negative for any known medical conditions. She has never been hospitalized and has no known drug allergies. Her immunizations are up to date for her age, including an influenza vaccine 3 months ago. She began her menses about a year ago. She is in the ninth grade at a public school and an average student. She states, "Everybody at school is sick."

Allergies

No known drug allergies; no known food allergies.

Medications

- Acetaminophen 325 mg tablets—two every 4 to 6 hours PRN. Last dose was 4 hours ago.
- An OTC cough medicine she does not recall the name of. The mother thinks it is a generic Robitussin DM. It is not helping.

Physical Examination

- *Vitals:* T 39.0°C (102.2°F), P 102, R 24, BP 120/76, SpO_2 95% on room air, WT 58 kg (129 lb), HT 165 cm (65 in.), BMI 21.5 (about 75th percentile).
- *General:* Ill appearing with frequent coughing but no acute distress.
- *Psychiatric:* Normal mood and affect.
- *Eyes:* Sclerae clear.
- *ENT/Mouth:* Nasal mucosa shows boggy edema with scant mucopurulent drainage bilaterally. Mouth mucosa pink and moist with mild posterior pharyngeal erythema. There is no sinus tenderness to facial percussion.
- *Neck:* Supple with firm, mobile, and fingertip-sized BL nontender lymphadenopathy.

- *Lungs:* No accessory muscle use with good air movement. There are diffuse moist rhonchi and end-expiratory wheezes at the bases. There is dullness to percussion in the lower lung fields.
- *Heart:* RRR, with normal S1 and S2. No murmurs, rubs, or gallops.
- *Abdomen:* Normal BS, soft and nontender; no organomegaly.
- *Neurologic:* A&O×3.

CLINICAL DISCUSSION QUESTIONS

1. What is the differential diagnosis?

2. What is the most likely diagnosis? Why?

3. Demonstrate your understanding about the pathophysiology of the most likely diagnosis.

4. Should tests/imaging studies be ordered? Which ones? Why? Think about tests/imaging beyond the primary care setting as well.

5. What are the next appropriate steps in management?

6. What is the prevalence in this patient population? What are the diagnostic challenges and treatment options for this diagnosis? Provide references for your responses.

7. What are the pertinent ICD-10 and CPT (E/M) codes for this visit? Provide a short rationale.

8. What is the appropriate patient education topic for this case?

9. If not managed appropriately, what is/are the medical/legal concern(s) that may arise?

10. Think about interprofessional collaboration for this case. Provide a list of specialties or other disciplines and indicate what contribution these professionals might make to managing the patient.

Bedside Manner Questions

11. What would your communication style/approach be with this patient and her mother?

12. If a patient and her mother are distressed by the diagnosis, what might offer support?

Answers available at courseconnect.springerpub.com.

HEADACHE AND FEVER, PEDIATRIC MALE

CASE 67

Chief Complaint

"Headache and fever."

History of Present Illness

An 8-year-old boy is brought to his pediatric office for a rapidly worsening headache and fever. Parents report he had been in a good state of health and returned about 5 days ago from a week at a scout camp. They deny any recent head injury. There have been no known tick bites. On the last day of camp, he began to feel tired and developed a headache and fever. The maximum fever they obtained at home was (39.5°C) 103.2°F. His appetite has been steadily declining over the past 10 hours or so. They tried ibuprofen, and it helped the headache initially but no longer seems to give relief. He denies cough, congestion, sore throat, diarrhea, or rash. He has vomited once in the past 30 minutes. Over the past 2 hours, he has not been himself. He does not want to move, wants the lights out, and is less interactive. He moans and complains of head and neck pain. The nurse informs the PCP that the boy is not speaking clearly when she asks him questions and he is confused. She has tried to find out where his headache is localized, but he cannot offer that information at this time. He cannot explain severity either. The nurse feels this patient requires immediate attention.

Review of Systems

His ROS was positive for headache, fever, confusion, neck pain, vomiting, anorexia, and nausea. His ROS is negative for cough, congestion, sore throat, rash, or diarrhea. He denies dysuria, hematuria, and abdominal pain. No wheezing or SOB is noted.

Relevant History

Patient has a history of exercise-induced asthma that is well controlled with the use of his albuterol inhaler prior to activities. He takes no other medication or supplements. He has no prior surgery history. He has no allergies to medication, and his vaccinations are up to date. He lives with his mother and father in an apartment that was built in the last 5 years. His only recent travel was the scout camp. The paternal history is positive for IBS. The maternal history is positive for hypothyroidism diagnosed at the age of 21.

Allergies

No known drug allergies; no known food allergies.

Medications

Albuterol inhaler 1 to 2 puffs inhaled X1: start 5 to 30 minutes before exercise.

Physical Examination

- *Vitals:* T 40°C (104°F), P 115, R 22, BP 102/68, WT 30.2 kg (66.5 lb), HT 137.2 cm (54 in.), BMI 16.
- *General:* Ill appearing. Moans and cries at times. Answers some questions but seems confused about where he currently is.

- *Skin, Hair, and Nails:* Warm and dry. Few scattered petechiae are noted on the lower extremities that were not noted in nurse documentation. These lesions are not blanchable. No peripheral edema. No jaundice. No abnormal findings with hair and nail exam.
- *Head:* Normocephalic. Atraumatic with no bruising noted.
- *Eyes:* Refuses eye exam and cries, "The light is too bright." Pupils appear equal and reactive. Cannot assess extraocular muscles at this time.
- *ENT/Mouth:* TMs are pearly bilaterally with no erythema or effusion. Nares are patent with no congestion. Oropharynx is somewhat dry but without erythema or exudate.
- *Neck:* Very tender to palpation. Patient refuses to bend neck forward and cries in pain if attempted. Flexion at the hips occurs when forcibly attempted. This is noted as a positive Brudzinski sign. Mild scattered anterior cervical adenopathy. Nodes mobile and not firm. No thyromegaly.
- *Lungs:* CTA bilaterally. No wheezes or crackles. Good aeration noted throughout. No stridor.
- *Heart:* RRR with no murmur noted.
- *Abdomen:* Soft. Cries with palpation but does not localize to a single area. No rebound. No guarding. BS normal throughout all fields. Nondistended.
- *Genital/Rectal:* Normal Tanner 1 on exam. Rectal exam deferred.
- *Musculoskeletal:* Patient is noncooperative for thorough exam. Will not stand up from bed for exam secondary to neck pain and headache. Muscle strength appears equal in the upper and lower extremities bilaterally at likely 4/5. Attempts to move hips in to a flexed position and then extend the lower legs while laying flat are met with intense resistance and moans of pain. This is a positive Kernig sign.
- *Neurologic:* Patient is noncooperative for thorough exam. Will not stand up from bed for exam secondary to neck pain and headache. Will not cooperate to check CNs secondary to pain in the neck and head; appear intact. Attempts to check deep tendon reflexes are met with cries when he has to move. Incomplete exam but appears to have reflexes of +3/5 in the upper and lower extremities that are symmetric.

CLINICAL DISCUSSION QUESTIONS

1. What is the differential diagnosis?

____

____

____

____

2. What is the most likely diagnosis? Why?

____

____

____

____

3. Demonstrate your understanding about the pathophysiology of the most likely diagnosis.

4. Should tests/imaging studies be ordered? Which ones? Why? Think about tests/imaging beyond the primary care setting as well.

5. What are the next appropriate steps in management?

6. What are physical exam findings, treatment approach, causes, and prevention of the diagnosis? Provide references for your response.

7. What are the pertinent ICD-10 and CPT (E/M) codes for this visit? Provide a short rationale.

8. What is the appropriate patient education topic for this case?

9. If not managed appropriately, what is/are the medical/legal concern(s) that may arise?

10. Think about possible interprofessional collaboration in this case. Provide a list of specialties or other disciplines and indicate what contribution these professionals might make to managing the patient.

BEDSIDE MANNER QUESTIONS

11. What would your communication style/approach be with this patient and his parents?

12. If a patient and his parents are distressed by the diagnosis, what might offer support?

Answers available at courseconnect.springerpub.com.

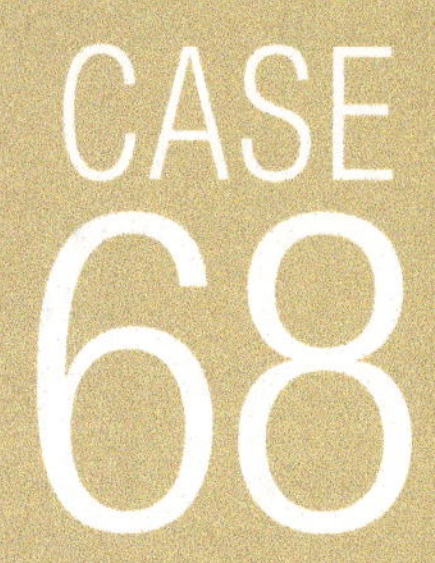

DOUBLE AND BLURRED VISION, ADOLESCENT MALE

Chief Complaint

"Double and blurred vision."

History of Present Illness

A 15-year-old boy, accompanied by his mother, presents to a new PCP with a 2-week history of double and blurred vision. He has not had any prior episodes. He reports he first noticed it during physical education class. The episodes last about 5 to 10 minutes each time. Over the past 2 weeks, he recalls having about 10 episodes. He reports that resting relieves his symptoms. They tend to be worse the longer he is physically active or if he is having a particularly stressful day. He reports having occasional headaches; however, he denies headache currently. When the headaches occur, he describes them as throbbing with pain behind both eyes. He denies SOB and chest pain.

Review of Systems

The patient's ROS is positive for fatigue, double and blurred vision, and occasional headaches. He denies current headache or vision changes. The patient reported past dizziness and light headedness; he has not had any syncope. He denies being dizzy at the time of exam. His ROS is negative for fever, chills, palpitations, heat or cold intolerance, SOB, edema, or chest pain. His weight has been stable, and he denies any heat or cold intolerance.

Relevant History

The patient's history is positive for obesity. His mother reports that previous health providers had expressed concern about his elevated BP. She does not recall the BP readings but was told they were elevated on more than one occasion. According to previous healthcare providers, he attempted lifestyle changes but failed. The patient has no other medical history. His immunizations are up to date. He lives with his parents and 7-year-old sister. He reports enjoying school; he is a sophomore and enjoys reading and hanging out with his friends. He has a relatively sedentary lifestyle; he exercises only when required in his gym class. His family history is positive for his mother with HTN and T2DM; his father has hyperlipidemia and reports having "borderline" high BP. His sister is healthy. Maternal grandparents are unknown; his mother was adopted. Paternal grandfather is deceased but had a history of stroke, MI, and HTN; he passed away from a second stroke at age 60. Paternal grandmother, age 73, is alive and with obesity, HTN, T2DM, and hyperlipidemia.

Allergies

No known drug allergies; no known food allergies.

Medications

None.

Physical Examination

- *Vitals:* T 36.7°C (98.2°F); P 90; R 16; BP 138/86; HT 175.26 cm (69 in.), ~75th percentile for age; WT 80.164 kg (180 lb); BMI 26.6, 95th percentile for his age.
- *General:* Appears calm in no acute distress. Obese, appears to be stated age.
- *Psychiatric:* Calm and cooperative.

- *Skin, Hair, and Nails:* Skin intact, no tenting or rashes noted. No abnormal findings with hair or nails.
- *Head:* Normocephalic, no deformities noted.
- *Eyes:* PERRLA. Vision 20/20 with both eyes.
- *Neck:* Supple, FROM, no thyromegaly noted.
- *Lungs:* CTA in all lung fields.
- *Heart:* RRR. No murmurs, rubs, or gallops noted.
- *Musculoskeletal:* FROM in all extremities, no edema or deformities noted.
- *Neurologic:* The patient is alert, attentive, and oriented. Speech is clear and fluent.
- *Cranial nerves:* II—Visual fields are full to confrontation; funduscopic exam is normal with sharp discs and no vascular changes; pupils are 4 mm and briskly reactive to light; visual acuity is 20/20 bilaterally. III, IV, VI—There is no eye deviation; convergence is impaired; PERRLA. V—Facial sensation is intact; corneal reflexes are intact. VII—Face is symmetric. VIII—Hearing is normal to rubbing fingers and whisper test. IX, X—Palate elevates symmetrically; phonation is normal. XI—Head turning and shoulder shrug are intact. XII—Tongue is midline with normal movements and no atrophy. Motor: There is no pronator drift of out-stretched arms; no atrophy noted; strength 5/5 bilaterally. Reflexes: 2+ and symmetric in the bilateral upper and lower extremities; sensory is intact bilaterally. Coordination: There are no abnormal or extraneous movements; Romberg is negative. Gait/stance: Posture is normal; gait is steady.

CLINICAL DISCUSSION QUESTIONS

1. What is the differential diagnosis?

___

___

___

___

2. What is the most likely diagnosis? Why?

___

___

___

___

3. Demonstrate your understanding about the pathophysiology of the most likely diagnosis.

___

___

___

___

4. Should tests/imaging studies be ordered? Which ones? Why? Think about tests/imaging beyond the primary care setting as well.

5. What are the next appropriate steps in management?

6. What are the risk factors, diagnostic criteria, and treatment options of the diagnosis? Provide references for your response.

7. What are the pertinent ICD-10 and CPT (E/M) codes for this visit? Provide a short rationale.

8. What is the appropriate patient education topic for this case?

9. If not managed appropriately, what is/are the medical/legal concern(s) that may arise?

10. Think about interprofessional collaboration for this case. Provide a list of specialties or other disciplines and indicate what contribution these professionals might make to managing the patient.

BEDSIDE MANNER QUESTION

11. What would be your communication style/approach with this patient and parent?

Answers available at courseconnect.springerpub.com.

CASE 69

IRREGULAR MENSTRUAL CYCLE, ADOLESCENT FEMALE

Chief Complaint

"Irregular menstrual cycle."

History of Present Illness

A 17-year-old young woman presents to her PCP with a 1-year history of irregular menses, including skipped menses, menorrhagia, and dysmenorrhea. She presents to the appointment with her mother, who assists as historian. She started menarche at age 14 and states she has never really had regular menses. Over the past year, menses have increased in irregularity and flow with clots and menstrual cramping. Menses are 7 days in length with mild to moderate clots. Patient uses tampons and changes them hourly for the first 3 to 4 days and then every 3 hours for the last 2 to 3 days of her menses. The patient states that she typically does not have a menses about twice a year, usually during a time of excess physical activity and stress.

Review of Systems

The patient's ROS is positive for nausea, abdominal pain (menstrual cramping), heavy menstrual flow, and intermittent dizziness. Her ROS is negative for decrease in appetite, weight change, hair loss, vaginal discharge, depression, or fatigue.

Relevant History

The patient has no history of depression or eating disorders and no history of chronic medical problems or surgery. She lives with parents and siblings in a single-family home. She takes advanced placement classes in school in the 12th grade at the local high school. The patient is active in school and community sports, including dance, volleyball, and soccer. She has been very involved with sports in middle and high school. Her family history is positive for thyroid disorders and HTN but negative for bleeding disorders. She denies being sexually active. She denies any eating disorder tendencies. She denies any usage of tobacco, alcohol, and drugs.

Allergies

No known drug allergies; no known food allergies.

Medications

None.

Physical Examination

- *Vitals:* T 37°C (98.7°F); P 98; R 22; BP 108/62; WT 55.34 kg (122 lb), 50th percentile; HT 165 cm (65 in.), 60th percentile; BMI 20.
- *General:* Appears mildly fatigued.
- *Psychiatric:* Affect is normal and appropriate.
- *Head:* Head is normocephalic. Hair distribution is normal without hair loss.
- *Eyes:* PERRL, red reflex present bilaterally. EOM full, positive nystagmus.
- *ENT/Mouth:* TMs pearly gray with visible cone of light and landmarks. Mucosa is pink and moist. Normal speech and tone. Uvula midline.
- *Neck:* Neck supple, no thyromegaly, or adenopathy.

- *Lungs:* Respirations even and unlabored, clear bilaterally.
- *Heart:* Normal S1 S2 without rubs, murmurs, or gallops.
- *Abdomen:* Soft, nontender, BS ×4, no organomegaly or splenomegaly. No costovertebral angle tenderness.
- *Musculoskeletal:* Moves all extremities well, equal strength, gait normal, DTRs 2+ bilaterally.
- *Neurological:* A&O×3, CN II to XII grossly intact. Sensory grossly intact to light touch symmetrically.

Clinical Discussion Questions

1. What is the differential diagnosis?

2. What is the most likely diagnosis? Why?

3. Demonstrate your understanding about the pathophysiology of the most likely diagnosis.

4. Should tests/imaging studies be ordered? Which ones? Why? Think about tests/imaging beyond the primary care setting as well.

5. What are the next appropriate steps in management?

6. Review a credible article(s) about environmental factors and characteristics of menarche associated with the diagnosis. Provide your references.

7. What are the pertinent ICD-10 and CPT (E/M) codes for this visit? Provide a short rationale.

8. What is the appropriate patient education topic for this case?

9. If not managed appropriately, what is/are the medical/legal concern(s) that may arise?

10. Think about interprofessional collaboration for this case. Provide a list of specialties or other disciplines and indicate what contribution these professionals might make to managing the patient.

Bedside Manner Questions

11. What would your communication style/approach be with this patient and mother?

12. If the patient and her mother are distressed by the diagnosis, what might offer support?

Answers available at courseconnect.springerpub.com.

CASE 70

BLOOD IN URINE, PEDIATRIC FEMALE

Chief Complaint

"Blood in urine."

History of Present Illness

A 7-year-old girl visited her regular PCP accompanied by her parents due to a recent onset of symptoms. Over the past 2 days, she experienced pain during urination, followed by the alarming presence of blood in her urine and the onset of fever. Her parents noted her discomfort during urination and observed her temperature peaking at 38.5°C (101.3°F). Additionally, they noticed her spending most of her time in bed due to overall discomfort and malaise. Concerned about the presence of blood in her urine, they sought medical attention. Initially, she found temporary relief with OTC acetaminophen, but the symptoms recurred despite the temporary improvement. Neither the parents nor the patient reported urinary frequency, unusual urine odor, urinary incontinence, nausea, vomiting, loss of appetite, back pain, flank pain, abdominal pain, or pain in the lower abdomen. The patient does not comprehend terms like "chills" or "nausea." This is the first instance of such symptoms, and there are no known structural abnormalities in the urinary tract according to the parents.

Review of Systems

The patient's ROS is positive for fever, dysuria, and hematuria. The patient's ROS is negative for weight loss, fatigue, night sweats, cough, SOB, chest pain, joint pain, joint swelling, headache, seizures, rhinorrhea, or sore throat.

Relevant History

The patient's history is unremarkable with no medical conditions reported. There are no known structural abnormalities in the urinary tract. She is up to date on all recommended immunizations. There is no surgical history or hospitalization history.

Allergies

No known drug allergies; no known food allergies.

Medications

Acetaminophen (160 mg / 5 mL) oral suspension 2.5 mL Q6h.

Physical Examination

- *Vitals:* T 38.8°C (101.8°F), P 96, RR 14, BP 96/68 mm Hg, HT 121 cm (47.6 in), WT 22.6 kg (51 lb), BMI 15.8.
- *General:* Appears conversant and uncomfortable.
- *Psychiatric:* A&O×3 and engages in coherent conversation.
- *Skin, Hair, and Nails:* Skin is pale and slightly flushed, with no rash or visible lesions. Nails appear smooth without evidence of hemorrhage.
- *Lungs:* CTA bilaterally. No wheezes, rales, or rhonchi.
- *Heart:* RRR, without murmur or gallop.

- *Abdomen:* Soft and flat, BS were normoactive across all quadrants. No guarding or rebound tenderness. Mild suprapubic discomfort on palpation. No tenderness to palpation in the umbilical region, RLQ, or LLQ. No costovertebral angle tenderness bilaterally.
- *Genital/Rectal:* Normal female genitalia, SMR 1.

CLINICAL DISCUSSION QUESTIONS

1. What is the differential diagnosis?

2. What is the most likely diagnosis? Why?

3. Demonstrate your understanding about the pathophysiology of the most likely diagnosis.

4. Should tests/imaging studies be ordered? Which ones? Why? Think about tests/imaging beyond the primary care setting as well.

5. What are the next appropriate steps in management?

6. What are the diagnostic approach, treatment options, and clinical presentation of the diagnosis? Provide references for your response.

7. What are the pertinent ICD-10 and CPT (E/M) codes for this visit? Provide a short rationale.

8. What is the appropriate patient education topic for this case?

9. If not managed appropriately, what is/are the medical/legal concern(s) that may arise?

10. Think about interprofessional collaboration for this case. Provide a list of specialties or other disciplines and indicate what contribution these professionals might make to managing the patient.

BEDSIDE MANNER QUESTION

11. What would your communication style/approach be with this patient?

Answers available at courseconnect.springerpub.com.

CASE 71

CHEST PAIN, ADOLESCENT MALE

Chief Complaint

"Chest pain."

History of Present Illness

A 14-year-old otherwise healthy boy presents with his mother to his PCP complaining of right-sided chest pain, which began 1 day ago after he sustained an injury. The patient states he was playing tackle football with friends when he received an injury to the right side of his chest from a player's elbow. He immediately fell to the ground in pain. He lay still for 1 to 2 minutes, expecting the pain to subside, but it did not. He attempted to continue playing but experienced difficulty taking a deep breath and the pain was more noticeable when running and twisting. The patient took 600 mg of ibuprofen the night before, but the medication did not relieve his pain. After a restless night, his mother has brought him for evaluation.

Review of Systems

The patient's ROS is positive for SOB, chest pain, decreased ROM of torso due to pain, and bruising after an injury. The patient is negative for fever, vision changes, loss of consciousness, cough, palpitations, edema, nausea, vomiting, diarrhea, numbness, and tingling.

Relevant History

The boy's medical history is unremarkable. His immunizations are up to date, he has no surgical history, and he takes no medications. He lives with his mother, father, and 10-year-old sister. He denies alcohol, tobacco, or illicit drug use. The family history is noncontributory.

Allergies

No known drug allergies; no known food allergies.

Medications

Ibuprofen 600 mg PRN for pain.

Physical Examination

- *Vitals:* T 37.7°C (99.8°F), P 102, R 24, BP 124/76, SpO_2 98%, WT 61.90 kg (136.5 lb), HT 162.5 cm (64 in.), BMI 23.6.
- *General:* Appears in acute distress.
- *Psychiatric:* Mildly anxious.
- *Skin, Hair, and Nails:* No rash; skin warm and dry. No abnormal findings with hair or nails.
- *Chest:* Bruising and tenderness to palpation of right lateral chest wall located in mid-axillary line at approximately the 4th and 5th intercostal spaces. No pain with lateral rotation of torso. Pain elicited with forward flexion and extension of the torso. Symmetrical movement of chest wall with inspiration and expiration.
- *Lungs:* CTA bilaterally with diminished BS in right lower lobe. Percussion to posterior chest wall on right demonstrates hyperresonance.
- *Heart:* RRR; no murmurs, rubs, or gallops.

- *Abdomen:* Soft, nontender, nondistended. No hepatosplenomegaly. Positive BS in all four quadrants.
- *Neurologic:* A&O×3, with no focal motor or sensory deficits noted.

CLINICAL DISCUSSION QUESTIONS

1. What is the differential diagnosis?

2. What is the most likely diagnosis? Why?

3. Demonstrate your understanding about the pathophysiology of to the most likely diagnosis.

4. Should tests/imaging studies be ordered? Which ones? Why? Think about tests/imaging beyond the primary care setting as well.

5. What are the next appropriate steps in management?

6. Review a reliable and recent article and discuss the treatment approach for this diagnosis. Include the reference.

7. What are the pertinent ICD-10 and CPT (E/M) codes for this visit? Provide a short rationale.

8. What is the appropriate patient education topic for this case?

9. If not managed appropriately, what is/are the medical/legal concern(s) that may arise?

10. Think about interprofessional collaboration for this case. Provide a list of specialties or other disciplines and indicate what contribution these professionals might make to managing the patient.

BEDSIDE MANNER QUESTIONS

11. What would your communication style/approach be with this patient and his mother?

12. If a patient and his mother are distressed by the diagnosis, what might offer support?

____

____

____

____

Answers available at courseconnect.springerpub.com.

UNSTEADY GAIT AND NAUSEA, PEDIATRIC FEMALE

CASE 72

Chief Complaint

"Unsteady gait and nausea."

History of Present Illness

A 6-year-old girl is brought by her father for evaluation of an unsteady gait. Her symptoms began 3 hours ago. The child's father was initially concerned that she "might be coming down with something again" because she asked to be carried downstairs after waking up and chose to watch television before breakfast instead of playing with her siblings like she usually does. When she got up from the couch, her father noted that she walked with her feet far apart and seemed to sway to the right side. The child states her head "felt weird and heavy" when she walked and that the sensation was worse when she moved her head, "like after I spin around on my dad's office chair." Her father also states that she does not seem to be hearing well. She vomited shortly after walking back to the couch. There is no report of recent falls or injuries and no new physical activities. The child denies headache, back pain, or leg pain and reports no numbness or weakness in her legs or feet. She was in the office last week and was diagnosed with a viral URI. The PCP recommended symptomatic treatment with nasal saline. She has been asymptomatic for the past 4 days. Currently, there are no sick contacts at home or in her class at school.

Review of Systems

The child's ROS is positive for nausea, vomiting, dizziness, unsteady gait, and decreased hearing on the right side. Her ROS is negative for fever, headache, cough, abdominal pain, diarrhea, constipation, eye pain, vision changes, rhinorrhea, ear pain, throat pain, upper or lower extremity pain, joint pain or swelling, numbness, or weakness.

Medical History

The child had a tonsillectomy at age 5. Her immunizations are up to date including annual influenza vaccine. She lives with parents and two siblings (ages 4 and 9) with whom she plays well. She entered first grade this year and performs well in class. She has multiple friends at school. She eats three meals per day along with an afternoon snack. She often still takes a 1-hour afternoon nap. She participates in soccer and dance classes on alternating weekends. Her parents and siblings have no significant medical history.

Allergies

No known drug allergies; no known food allergies.

Medications

None.

Physical Examination

- *Vitals:* T 37°C (98.6°F), P 82, R 20, BP 96/58, WT 20 kg (44 lb), HT 115 cm (45.28 in), BMI 15.1 (47th percentile).
- *General:* Well dressed/well groomed, smiles, is talkative, sits very still in chair.
- *Skin, Hair, and Nails:* Skin warm and dry, no rashes, lesions, bruising, or discoloration. No abnormal findings with hair or nails.

- *Head:* Normocephalic, nontender, and atraumatic.
- *Eyes:* PERRLA, EOMI, spontaneous left-beating horizontal nystagmus that resolves with fixation.
- *ENT/Mouth:* Ear canal clear, TMs visible bilaterally without erythema or effusion, nares patent, turbinates pink and moist, good oral hygiene, and oropharynx mucosa pink and moist.
- *Heart:* RRR, no murmurs, brisk capillary refill, no cyanosis, distal pulses intact.
- *Lungs:* CTA bilaterally, chest wall movement adequate and symmetrical, no retractions or use of accessory muscles.
- *Abdomen:* BS active in all quadrants, soft, nontender, nondistended.
- *Musculoskeletal:* Ambulates without aid but waivers right when walking straight, no scoliosis or spinal abnormalities, FROM upper and lower extremities, good muscle tone, strength 5/5 upper and lower extremities.
- *Neurologic:* A&O×3, CN to XII grossly intact, except hearing decreased on right with whisper test (VIII), DTR (patellar and Achilles tendon) 2+ bilaterally.

Clinical Discussion Questions

1. What is the differential diagnosis?

____

____

____

____

2. What is the most likely diagnosis? Why?

____

____

____

____

3. Demonstrate your understanding about the pathophysiology of the most likely diagnosis.

____

____

____

____

4. Should tests/imaging studies be ordered? Which ones? Why? Think about tests/imaging beyond the primary care setting as well.

____

____

____

____

5. What are the next appropriate steps in management?

6. What is the prevalence and what are the treatment options for this diagnosis? Provide references for your response.

7. What are the pertinent ICD-10 and CPT (E/M) codes for this visit? Provide a short rationale.

8. What is the appropriate patient education topic for this case?

9. If not managed appropriately, what is/are the medical/legal concern(s) that may arise?

10. Think about interprofessional collaboration for this case. Provide a list of specialties or other disciplines and indicate what contribution these professionals might make to managing the patient.

Bedside Manner Question

11. What would your communication style/approach be with this patient and parent?

Answers available at courseconnect.springerpub.com.

CASE 73

EXCESS FACIAL HAIR, ADOLESCENT FEMALE

Chief Complaint

"Excessive facial hair."

History of Present Illness

An unaccompanied 16-year-old girl presents to her PCP complaining of excessive facial hair and acne. Her symptoms have increased gradually over the last 2 to 3 years along with a 60-lb weight gain since her last visit 2 years ago. The reason for this visit is distress that her acne and dark facial hair are causing social problems for her. She requests isotretinoin that was helpful for a friend.

The patient is less concerned about her weight but states she has tried to lose weight without success. She snacks frequently and has switched from "donuts and candy to protein bars" without success. She denies laxative use or induction of vomiting. She drinks six to 12 diet sodas daily. The patient is an only child and both parents often work late, leaving her frozen dinners. She avoids gym class whenever possible and does not exercise. She admits to some depressed mood and does not think her prescribed fluoxetine has helped her, but she continues to take it at her parents' request.

She denies current or past sexual activity. Menarche began age 11 with her periods regular at age 12, then gradually becoming lighter and less frequent over the past 3 years. Her periods now last 2 to 3 days and occur every 6 to 8 weeks. She is a long-time patient of the clinic, last seen 2 years ago for a well-child visit. At that time, she was diagnosed with situational (school-related) depression and acne. She was prescribed fluoxetine 20 mg QD and clindamycin 1% lotion BID. Refills are charted for the fluoxetine but not the clindamycin. Her chart contains a blanket permission from her parents to see the patient unaccompanied and she also brings a note to that effect today.

Review of Systems

The patient's ROS is positive for sleeping 9 to 10 hours most nights and expressing some guilt about overeating sweets. Her ROS is negative for polydipsia, polyuria, polyphagia, hair loss, change in skin color or texture or thickening of facial features, tremor, palpitations, diarrhea, constipation, or suicidal or homicidal ideation.

Relevant History

The patient is current on all vaccinations, including HPV. She is of mixed White and Black ancestry and states other family members are not as hairy as she. She is interested in boys but has not started dating or engaged in any romantic or sexual interaction. She denies smoking, alcohol, or drug use.

Allergies

No known drug allergies; no known food allergies.

Medications

Fluoxetine 20 mg QD for depressed mood.

Physical Examination

- *Vitals:* T 37.1°C (98.8°F), P 80, R 14, BP 130/82, HT 165.3 cm (65 in.), WT 80.74 kg (178 lb), BMI 29.6.
- *General:* Talkative female in no acute distress.
- *Psychiatric:* A&O×3 with appropriate mood and affect.

- *Skin, Hair, and Nails:* Acne on face and upper chest and back; oily skin with papules, comedones, pustules. Mild hirsutism of face and forearms. No alopecia. No thickening or darkening of skin.
- *Head:* Normocephalic, atraumatic.
- *Eyes:* PERRL, EOMI.
- *ENT/Mouth:* Nares patent, turbonates clear; TMs without erythema or effusion; dentition with multiple fillings and caries.
- *Chest:* Symmetric excursion with no accessory muscle use.
- *Lungs:* Resonant with vesicular breath sounds all fields, no wheezes, rales, or rhonchi.
- *Heart:* Quiet precordium, RSR, no murmur, rub, or gallop.
- *Abdomen:* Protuberant, NABS in all quadrants, no bruit, nontender, no masses, no costovertebral angle tenderness.
- *Genital/Rectal:* Deferred.
- *Musculoskeletal:* FROM and 5/5 strength in all extremities.
- *Neurological:* Gait smooth, no tremor or past pointing.

CLINICAL DISCUSSION QUESTIONS

1. What is the differential diagnosis?

2. What is the most likely diagnosis? Why?

3. Demonstrate your understanding about the pathophysiology of the most likely diagnosis.

4. Should tests/imaging studies be ordered? Which ones? Why? Think about tests/imaging beyond the primary care setting as well.

5. What are the next appropriate steps in management?

6. What is the diagnostic and management approach with this condition in adolescent patients? Provide references for your response.

7. What are the pertinent ICD-10 and CPT (E/M) codes for this visit? Provide a short rationale.

8. What is the appropriate patient education topic for this case?

9. If not managed appropriately, what is/are the medical/legal concern(s) that may arise?

10. Think about interprofessional collaboration for this case. Provide a list of specialties or other disciplines and indicate what contribution these professionals might make to managing the patient.

BEDSIDE MANNER QUESTION

11. What would your communication style/approach be with this patient?

Answers available at courseconnect.springerpub.com.

FEVER, COUGH, AND RUNNY NOSE, PEDIATRIC FEMALE

CASE 74

Chief Complaint

"Fever, cough, and runny nose."

History of Present Illness

During the summer season, a mother brings her 9-month-old daughter to her PCP for evaluation of fever, cough, and runny nose for the past week. The mother states her child's fever started off at 37.8°C (100°F), but for the past 2 days, it has been fluctuating between 38°C to 39°C (102°F to 103°F). She has been alternating between acetaminophen and ibuprofen every 4 to 6 hours. This brings the fever to 38.3°C (101°F). A dry intermittent cough has been present for the past 4 days and is negative for post-tussive emesis. Her runny nose has progressively been getting worse over the past 7 days and the discharge is green. She has a poor appetite but is drinking normally. The mother has not noticed the child pulling her ears or showing any discomfort with urination. There is no history of vomiting or diarrhea.

Review of Systems

The child's ROS is positive for fever, cough, runny nose, and a decrease in appetite. The ROS is negative for vomiting and diarrhea.

Relevant History

The child was born by NSVD, without any complications. She is up to date with immunizations, including influenza vaccines. The child lives with her parents, has two siblings, and attends daycare. Her father is a smoker but smokes away from the house and the car. Family history includes father being prediabetic and mother is obese.

Allergies

No known drug allergies; no known food allergies.

Medications

- Acetaminophen 160/5 mL 1 tsp Q4h PRN.
- Ibuprofen 100/5 mL 1 tsp Q6h PRN.

Physical Examination

- *Vitals:* T 39.3°C (102.7°F); P 130; R 28; BP 98/62; WT 10 kg (22 lb), 75th percentile; HT 68.6 cm (27 in.), 50th percentile; BMI 21.2.
- *General:* Slightly uncomfortable but aware of her surroundings. Not toxic.
- *Skin, Hair, and Nails:* Warm and pink. No abnormal findings with hair or nails.
- *ENT/Mouth:* Right TM: bulging, dull red, landmarks not visible. Left TM: slightly pink with a positive light reflex. Nose: purulent drainage. OP: patent and moist.
- *Lungs:* Coarse breath sounds, mostly transmitted from upper airway congestion. Negative for wheezing or rhonchi.
- *Heart:* RRR. No murmur was appreciated.

- *Abdomen:* Soft, nontender, nondistended.
- *Neurologic:* Alert and interactive.

CLINICAL DISCUSSION QUESTIONS

1. What is the differential diagnosis?

2. What is the most likely diagnosis? Why?

3. Demonstrate your understanding about the pathophysiology of the most likely diagnosis.

4. Should tests/imaging studies be ordered? Which ones? Why? Think about tests/imaging beyond the primary care setting as well.

5. What are the next appropriate steps in management?

6. What are the prevalence, prevention, risk factors, and treatments of the diagnosis? Provide the references for your responses.

7. What are the pertinent ICD-10 and CPT (E/M) codes for this visit? Provide a short rationale.

8. What is the appropriate patient education topic for this case?

9. If not managed appropriately, what is/are the medical/legal concern(s) that may arise?

10. Think about interprofessional collaboration for this case. Provide a list of specialties or other disciplines and indicate what contribution these professionals might make to managing the patient.

BEDSIDE MANNER QUESTION

11. What would your communication style/approach be with this parent?

Answers available at courseconnect.springerpub.com.

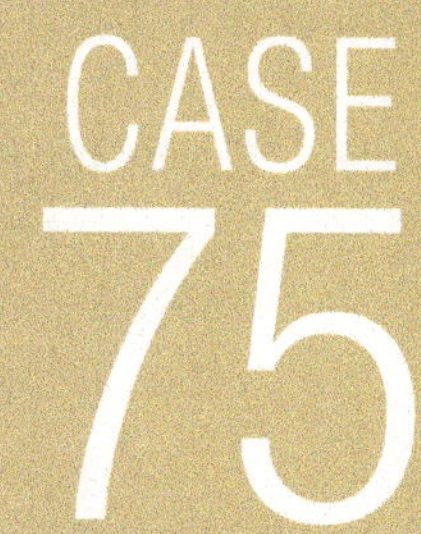

CASE 75

ABDOMINAL PAIN, ADOLESCENT MALE

Chief Complaint

"Abdominal pain."

History of Present Illness

A 17-year-old boy presents to his PCP with abdominal pain, nausea, vomiting, poor appetite, headache, and diarrhea. He has been sick since last night. He describes his abdominal pain as "really bad" and rates his pain level as 5/10. He states, "I don't know how to describe the pain, but I know it's really bad." He points to the entire abdomen as the location of the pain. When asked where the pain started, he states, "the whole stomach." He vomited once this afternoon and is now nauseous. He states he had loose stool this morning. He indicates that "most likely it was diarrhea this morning; but I am not 100% sure." He further states, "I do have loose stools a lot." He denies fever, chills, cough, runny nose, sore throat, abdominal bloating, acid reflux, neck stiffness, urinary urgency, dysuria, hematochezia, back pain, wheezing, SOB, recent travel, new medication, or known sick contacts at home or school. He does not recall eating or drinking anything out of ordinary and has been consuming essentially the same food and drinks as his entire family. He has been taking acetaminophen 500 mg every 6 hours to manage his pain, and it has helped his pain slightly. He is here today with his older sister, who drove him to the appointment.

Review of Systems

His ROS is positive for abdominal pain, nausea, and vomiting. He reports headache and lack of appetite. The ROS is questionable for diarrhea. The ROS is negative for fever, chills, constipation, cough, runny nose, sore throat, abdominal bloating, acid reflux, neck stiffness, urinary urgency, dysuria, hematochezia, back pain, wheezing, SOB, or chest pain.

Relevant History

The patient's medical history is significant for acne (onset age 14), obesity, hepatic steatosis, and mild intermittent asthma (onset age 8). He has no surgical history. His social history includes playing football and traveling with his family. He has two sisters and two brothers. He lives with his father and does not have much interaction with his mom. He has been sexually active since age 16 with one female partner. He uses condoms. His family history includes DM (paternal grandparents), HTN (father), and prostate cancer (paternal grandfather). He does not know his maternal family history.

Allergies

No known drug allergies; no known food allergies.

Medications

- Benzoyl peroxide 4% topical QD.
- Albuterol inhaler 2 puffs every 4 to 6 hours PRN.

PHYSICAL EXAMINATION

- *Vitals:* T 37.5°C (99.5°F), P 93, R 19, BP 130/87, WT 95.25 kg (210 lb), HT 177.8 cm (70 in.), BMI 30.1.
- *General:* Mild to moderate distress, obese.
- *Psychiatric:* Cooperative, appropriate mood and affect.
- *Eyes:* Conjunctiva and sclera clear.
- *ENT/Mouth:* Within normal limit.
- *Neck:* Supple, FROM.
- *Lungs:* CTA bilaterally.
- *Heart:* Normal rate, regular rhythm, no heart murmur.
- *Abdomen:* Tender abdomen throughout; greatest tenderness in RLQ—guarding even with mild palpation; McBurney point tenderness noted; psoas sign +; Rovsing sign questionable.
- *Neurologic:* A&O×3.

CLINICAL DISCUSSION QUESTIONS

1. What is the differential diagnosis?

2. What is the most likely diagnosis? Why?

3. Demonstrate your understanding about the pathophysiology of the most likely diagnosis.

4. Should tests/imaging studies be ordered? Which ones? Why? Think about tests/imaging beyond the primary care setting as well.

5. What are the next appropriate steps in management?

6. Demonstrate your understanding of the prevalence, diagnostic criteria, and treatment options. Include a list of your reference(s).

7. What are the pertinent ICD-10 and CPT (E/M) codes for this visit? Provide a short rationale.

8. What is the appropriate patient education topic for this case?

9. If not managed appropriately, what is/are the medical/legal concern(s) that may arise?

10. Think about interprofessional collaboration for this case. Provide a list of specialties or other disciplines and indicate what contribution these professionals might make to managing the patient.

BEDSIDE MANNER QUESTIONS

11. What would your communication style/approach be with this patient and his sister?

12. If a patient and his sister are distressed by the diagnosis, what might offer support?

Answers available at courseconnect.springerpub.com.

CASE 76

IRRITABLE AND CRYING TODDLER, PEDIATRIC MALE

Chief Complaint

"Irritable and crying toddler."

History of Present Illness

A mother presents with her 16-month-old son to his PCP for an evaluation of irritability and crying for the past 5 hours. According to his mother, the child was fine but suddenly became fussy and appeared to be in pain. He has no nausea, vomiting, diarrhea, fever, cough, or cold symptoms. His mother was alarmed by the sudden off-on episodes of crying. She explains that when he has short bursts of excruciating pain he doubles over or if he is being held his legs have pull up to his chest. The child seems to be fine in between these episodes. Typically, the child is calm.

Review of Systems

The patient's ROS is positive for irritability and possible abdominal pain. His ROS is negative for nausea, vomiting, bloody stool, constipation, fever, chills, and cough.

Relevant History

The child was an NSVD at term without any complications. He has continued to thrive, hitting all developmental milestones. He has not been hospitalized and he is not on any chronic medications.

Allergies

No known drug allergies; no known food allergies.

Medications

None.

Physical Examination

- *Vitals:* T 37.0°C (98.6°F); P 120; R 28; BP 100/65; WT 9.9 kg (22 lb), 10th percentile; HT 76.2 cm (30 in.), 5th percentile; BMI 16.5.
- *General:* Alert and engaging when not having an episode of pain. He is nontoxic looking.
- *Psychiatric:* Irritable.
- *Skin, Hair, and Nails:* Pink with a 1- to 2-second capillary refill. No abnormal findings with hair or nails.
- *Head:* No signs of trauma.
- *Eyes:* PERRL.
- *ENT/Mouth:* Moist oral mucosa with no signs of dehydration.
- *Neck:* FROM with no nuchal rigidity.
- *Lungs:* CTA bilaterally, equal breath sounds.
- *Heart:* RRR, no murmurs.
- *Abdomen:* Soft and nondistended. Mild tenderness with fullness in the right upper abdomen. The right lower abdomen is scaphoid and feels "empty" on palpation (dance sign).

- *Genital/Rectal:* Genital exam without abnormal finding; stool is hemoccult negative.
- *Neurologic:* Alert and not lethargic.

CLINICAL DISCUSSION QUESTIONS

1. What is the differential diagnosis?

2. What is the most likely diagnosis? Why?

3. Demonstrate your understanding about the pathophysiology of the most likely diagnosis.

4. Should tests/imaging studies be ordered? Which ones? Why? Think about tests/imaging beyond the primary care setting as well.

5. What are the next appropriate steps in management?

6. What is a cost-effective and highly specific diagnostic method for this diagnosis? What are the treatment options of this diagnosis? Provide references for your responses.

7. What are the pertinent ICD-10 and CPT (E/M) codes for this visit? Provide a short rationale.

8. What is the appropriate parent education topic for this case?

9. If not managed appropriately, what is/are the medical/legal concern(s) that may arise?

10. Think about interprofessional collaboration for this case. Provide a list of specialties or other disciplines and indicate what contribution these professionals might make to managing the patient.

BEDSIDE MANNER QUESTIONS

11. What would your communication style/approach be with this parent/patient?

12. If a patient's parent is distressed by the diagnosis, what might offer support?

Answers available at courseconnect.springerpub.com.

CASE 77

SWELLING AROUND EYES AND ANKLES, ADOLESCENT MALE

Chief Complaint

"Swelling around eyes and ankles."

History of Present Illness

A 16-year-old boy of Black and Filipino heritage arrives at his PCP office with his adoptive father for worsening swelling around his eyes and swollen ankles over the past week. He reports his eyes get puffy with seasonal allergies every fall, but they have never been this puffy. This morning, his feet were so swollen he could not put on shoes. He thought he had the stomach flu with loss of appetite, nausea, a couple of episodes of loose stool, and mild abdominal discomfort over the past week. He also states he has urinated only twice in the past 2 days. He has tried drinking more sports drink, but this has not helped. He works at a fast-food restaurant 3 evenings a week and admits French fries are a routine part of his diet. He plays on the school football team and has practice each day but wonders why he is so "out of shape" and exhausted. Today, he reports he is very tired, does not think he can participate in football practice, and is concerned his feet are too swollen for his cleats to fit.

Review of Systems

The patient's ROS is positive for loss of appetite; mild GI upset; nausea; loose stool; reduced urinary output, and significant swelling of eyelids and lips, torso, legs, and feet over the past couple of days. He also reports fatigue, poor exercise tolerance, and mild SOB over the past week. The ROS is negative for fever, chills, rashes, vomiting, constipation, dysuria, hematuria, sore throat, cough, chest pain, backache, injuries, or trauma.

Relevant History

The patient's history is limited due to adoption at age 3. His adoptive father reports typical childhood illnesses since his adoption, with eczema as a toddler and seasonal allergies since age 9. He has asthma with URIs and exercise-induced asthma, onset 1 year ago. No known illness or injuries are reported. He was seen for a sports clearance exam with this provider 9 weeks ago. He measured 157.48 cm (62 in.) and weighed 51.25 kg (113 lb). At that visit, urine dip was normal with only trace protein.

Before he was adopted, he was in foster care with an older sister for 2 years due to parental substance abuse. Perinatal drug exposure was suspected. His older biologic sister was adopted into another family and has a history of kidney transplant for unknown cause. He has no contact with his biologic parents or relatives. Adoptive parents have contact with the adoption agency and will seek more information about family and sibling medical history.

Allergies

No known drug allergies; no known food allergies.

Medications

- Albuterol HFA inhaler, 2 puffs 15 min pre-exercise and Q4h PRN for asthma.
- Naproxen sodium 220 mg PO, occasional use for post-sports-activity muscle aches.

Physical Examination

- *Vitals:* T 37°C (98.6°F), P 110, R 14, BP 122/62, SpO_2 98%, HT 157.48 cm (62 in.), WT 55.79 kg (123 lb), BMI 22.5. Note: 10 lb weight gain from exam 9 weeks prior.

- *General:* Mildly ill-appearing child alert and cooperative but with low energy.
- *Psychiatric:* Fatigued, mildly anxious, but nondepressed appearing.
- *Skin, Hair, and Nails:* Warm, dry, intact without rash; mild generalized swelling of trunk; mild edema of arms, moderate 3+ pitting edema lower extremities, especially ankles and feet, with moderate swelling extending into the scrotum.
- *Eyes:* PERRLA; eyes are narrowed to slits due to periorbital edema.
- *ENT/Mouth:* No lesions, posterior pharynx without erythema or exudate, uvula midline.
- *Neck:* No cervical lymphadenopathy, no JVD, mild generalized edema of face and neck.
- *Lungs:* CTA bilaterally.
- *Heart:* RRR; S1, S2 without murmur, gallop, or bruit.
- *Abdomen:* Mild distention with generalized edema, nontender, no hepatosplenomegaly, no costovertebral angle tenderness.
- *Genital/Rectal:* Generalized swelling into scrotum; no testicular lesions, warmth, redness, tenderness, or masses; no penile discharge. Rectal exam was deferred.
- *Neurologic:* A&O×3. CN II to XII grossly intact, appropriate verbal responses.
- *Office-Based Lab:* Urine dip SG 1.035, 3+ protein; negative glucose, blood, leukocytes, or nitrites. Note: urine dip on prior visit normal with only trace protein.

CLINICAL DISCUSSION QUESTIONS

1. What is the differential diagnosis?

____

____

____

____

2. What is the most likely diagnosis? Why?

____

____

____

____

3. Demonstrate your understanding about the pathophysiology of the most likely diagnosis.

____

____

____

____

4. Should tests/imaging studies be ordered? Which ones? Why? Think about tests/imaging beyond the primary care setting as well.

5. What are the next appropriate steps in management?

6. Review a reliable, recent reference and demonstrate an understanding of the initial and long-term management of this diagnosis. Provide references for your response.

7. What are the pertinent ICD-10 and CPT (E/M) codes for this visit? Provide a short rationale.

8. What is the appropriate patient education topic for this case?

9. If not managed appropriately, what is/are the medical/legal concern(s) that may arise?

10. Think about interprofessional collaboration for this case. Provide a list of specialties or other disciplines and indicate what contribution these professionals might make to managing the patient.

BEDSIDE MANNER QUESTIONS

11. What would your communication style/approach be with this patient and father?

12. If a patient and his adoptive father are distressed by the diagnosis, what might offer support?

Answers available at courseconnect.springerpub.com.

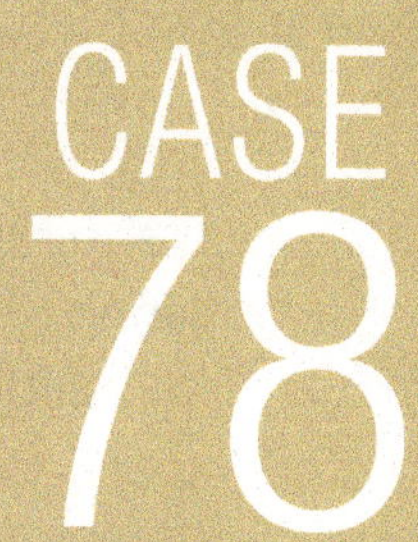

COUGHING AND GAGGING, PEDIATRIC MALE

Chief Complaint

"Coughing and gagging."

History of Present Illness

A mother brings her 3-month-old previously healthy infant to his PCP for evaluation of an apparent apnea episode that occurred that morning. He had developed a cough and nasal congestion about 5 days prior to this visit, and on the morning of the visit had a prolonged coughing spell followed by a gagging episode. His mother heard the cough and gagging over the baby monitor and when the gagging began, she ran to his room to check on him. By the time she picked him up from his crib, he did not seem to be breathing and his face and lips were blue. She immediately brought the baby to her husband, by which time the child had begun to breathe, and his color quickly returned to normal.

The episodes of cough have become more frequent and prolonged since the onset of the illness, but he has not had a fever. His mother reported she had been fighting off a "nagging cough" for about 3 weeks. The infant's 2-year-old sister and 4-year-old brother had no respiratory symptoms. None of the children attended day care.

Review of Systems

The infant's ROS is positive for decreased feeding and a few episodes of vomiting following coughing spells. The ROS is negative for fever, conjunctivitis, diarrhea, rash, or seizures.

Relevant History

The infant was born by vaginal delivery at 39 weeks' gestation following an uncomplicated pregnancy. His mother received regular prenatal care and had no history of untreated cervical infection. His birth weight was 6 lb 14 oz, and he was discharged home at 48 hours of age after an uneventful stay in the newborn nursery. He had an appropriate weight gain and normal development and physical examination at his 2-week, 1-month, and 2-month well-baby visits, and his routine newborn screening was normal. He had received all recommended immunizations, including those routinely administered at 2 months.

Allergies

No known drug allergies; no known food allergies.

Medications

None.

Physical Examination

- *Vitals:* T 37.1°C (98.8°F); P 140; R 40; BP 80/40; SpO_2 96%; HT 61 cm (24 in.), 43rd percentile; WT 5.5 kg (12 lb), 10th percentile; BMI 14.6.
- *General:* Alert and active, in no distress.
- *Skin, Hair, and Nails:* Acyanotic, no rash or lesions. No abnormal findings with hair or nails.
- *Head:* Anterior fontanelle soft and flat.
- *Eyes:* No discharge or conjunctival injection.

- *ENT/Mouth:* Nares congested, TMs clear, oral mucosa moist and without lesions.
- *Lungs:* CTA bilaterally, breath sounds equal bilaterally; no grunting, retractions, or nasal flaring.
- *Heart:* RRR, S1 and S2 normal intensity, no murmur, pulses 2+ in all extremities.
- *Abdomen:* Soft, no masses or hepatosplenomegaly.
- *Neurologic:* Alert, moving all extremities equally, normal muscle bulk and tone.

CLINICAL DISCUSSION QUESTIONS

1. What is the differential diagnosis?

2. What is the most likely diagnosis? Why?

3. Demonstrate your understanding about the pathophysiology of the most likely diagnosis.

4. Should tests/imaging studies be ordered? Which ones? Why? Think about tests/imaging beyond the primary care setting as well.

5. What are the next appropriate steps in management?

6. What are the preventive plans and treatment approaches for the diagnosis? Provide references for your response.

7. What are the pertinent ICD-10 and CPT (E/M) codes for this visit? Provide a short rationale.

8. What is the appropriate parent education topic for this case?

9. If not managed appropriately, what is/are the medical/legal concern(s) that may arise?

10. Think about interprofessional collaboration for this case. Provide a list of specialties or other disciplines and indicate what contribution these professionals might make to managing the patient.

BEDSIDE MANNER QUESTIONS

11. What would your communication style/approach be with this patient's mother?

12. If the patient's mother is distressed by the diagnosis, what might offer support?

Answers available at courseconnect.springerpub.com.

CASE 79

ASTHMA FOLLOW-UP, ADOLESCENT MALE

Chief Complaint

"Asthma follow-up."

History of Present Illness

A 13-year-old boy presents to a pediatrician for follow-up of long-standing asthma. He states that he gets tightness in his chest nearly every day, sometimes more than once a day. The episodes last for 5 to 10 minutes and cause him to stop his activities. He experiences no pain with the episodes. There is no pallor and his mother states that while he does not wheeze, he does breathe heavily but does not appear in respiratory distress. The patient states that during the episodes he is no more anxious "than someone who is having trouble with breathing." On further questioning, though, he states that he feels a great deal of stress and anxiety due to schoolwork and peer and family relationships. He repeatedly asks "Is that normal?" and "Am I okay?"

He is currently taking no medication since his albuterol inhaler ran out and was not refilled. When he does have the inhaler, he states that it helps his breathing and chest tightness. He takes an antihistamine OTC seasonally in the fall but is not currently taking it (in January).

The patient's mother reports that he "worries about every little thing." He complains of headaches several days per week, and his mother believes this is due to anxiety, which is also making focus at school difficult. She is not sure how long this has been going on, but it does seem to be getting worse recently. He usually sleeps well at night but has not been sleeping well recently—which he has attributed to the breathing issues.

Review of Systems

The patient has had no fevers and states he gets frequent headaches. He has seasonal allergies in the fall, but doesn't know the exact triggers. He gets stuffy and runny nose with allergy flares. No nosebleeds. Does not complain of sore throat nor hearing or vision difficulties.

He does not complain of chest pain, other than the tightness previously mentioned. He does not cough. He does occasionally wheeze, usually with respiratory infections, and is not sure whether he has wheezed with any of the current episodes.

He eats a normal diet and does not complain of constipation, diarrhea, nausea, or emesis. He occasionally complains of mild to moderate stomach aches, which resolve with drinking water and resting.

He has no musculoskeletal complaints. He does not complain of rash.

Relevant History

The patient was diagnosed with asthma at about age 7 but has had symptoms including wheezing with respiratory infections since a much younger age. He has averaged 2 ED visits per year, usually in the fall and winter, but has never required hospitalization. He has no surgical history.

During elementary school, he worked with a school counselor for some anxiety issues regarding his school work.

He denies smoking or vaping, and other than having witnessed others at school vaping in the rest room, he denies any environmental tobacco exposure. He feels safe in his home with no exposure to violence or abuse.

There is no family history of asthma, but mom and a sibling have allergic rhinitis. A maternal aunt has a diagnosed anxiety disorder.

Allergies

No known drug allergies; no known food allergies.

Medications

Albuterol inhaler PRN (not currently using).

Physical Examination

- *Vitals:* T 36.4°C (97.5°F; tympanic), P 100, R 18, BP 94/64, WT 65.7 kg (145 lb); Ht 170.2 cm (67 in.); BMI 22.7.
- *General:* Alert, interactive, and oriented x3, well appearing, in no acute distress.
- *Psychiatric:* GAD-7 Score is 14. The patient is alert, cooperative and candid. Anxious, with good insight and judgement and no suicidal or homicidal ideation. Some perseverance of speech around whether he was going crazy or might "go too far."
- *Skin, Hair, and Nails:* No rash or eczema.
- *Head:* Normocephalic, atraumatic, and without tenderness.
- *Eyes:* Conjunctiva and lids normal.
- *ENT/Mouth:* Ears—canals are patent and TMs are without erythema or effusion. Mouth—mucosa pink and moist, palate intact and tongue is normal.
- *Neck:* Supple with no lymphadenopathy.
- *Chest:* Nontender, no masses, no asymmetry.
- *Lungs:* No accessory muscle use, no retractions. Lungs were CTA and percussion bilaterally, symmetric air movement with no wheezes, rales, or rhonchi appreciated.
- *Heart:* RRR, S1 and S2 were audible with no murmur, pulses 2+ and symmetric, capillary refill <2 seconds, no cyanosis or clubbing.
- *Abdomen:* Soft, nontender, with no mass or organomegaly.
- *Neurologic:* No focal deficits, CN II to XII intact.

Clinical Discussion Questions

1. What is the differential diagnosis?

2. What is the most likely diagnosis? Why?

3. Demonstrate your understanding about the pathophysiology of the most likely diagnosis.

4. Should tests/imaging studies be ordered? Which ones? Why? Think about tests/imaging beyond the primary care setting as well.

5. What are the next appropriate steps in management?

6. What are the treatment options for this diagnosis? Provide references for your response.

7. What are the pertinent ICD-10 and CPT (E/M) codes for this visit? Provide a short rationale.

8. What is the appropriate patient education topic for this case?

9. If not managed appropriately, what is/are the medical/legal concern(s) that may arise?

10. Think about interprofessional collaboration for this case. Provide a list of specialties or other disciplines and indicate what contribution these professionals might make to managing the patient.

BEDSIDE MANNER QUESTION

11. How would you communicate your likely diagnosis to the patient and his mother?

Answers available at courseconnect.springerpub.com.

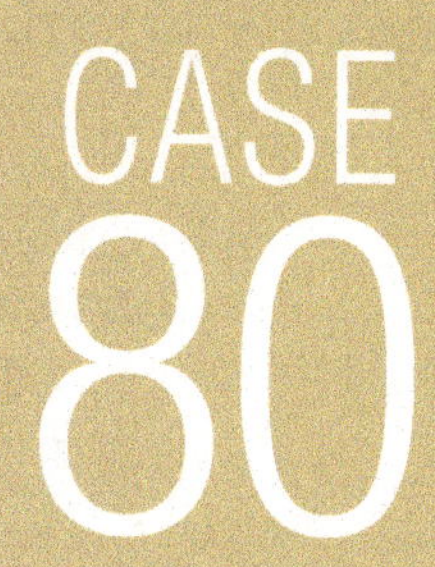

STOMACH PAIN AND BLOATING, ADOLESCENT FEMALE

Chief Complaint

"Stomach pain with bloating."

History of Present Illness

A 17-year-old young woman accompanied by her mother presents to her regular PCP with concerns of abdominal pain, bloating, and diarrhea over the past 6 months. The patient noticed worsening abdominal pain and diarrhea several days ago. She continues to have abdominal bloating and cramping with foul-smelling, watery diarrhea and flatus 7 days afterward. She tried bismuth subsalicylate and loperamide for diarrhea with little relief. She has missed multiple school days because of her abdominal pain and diarrhea. The patient has been on a lactose-free diet for 2 months with no improvement of her symptoms. She also stopped soft drinks and fast food. According to her mother, she has been more tired and moody for several months. Her last menstrual cycle was a week ago. She denies sexual activity for over 6 months and has had no recent travel.

Review of Systems

The patient's ROS is positive for unintentional weight loss of 10 lb, chronic fatigue, arthralgias, itchy rash on anterior lower legs, rhinorrhea, canker sores, abdominal pain, bloating, vomiting, occasional dyspepsia, persistent diarrhea, and moodiness. Her ROS is negative for fever, chills, nausea, changes in appetite, dysuria, pelvic pain, abnormal vaginal discharge or bleeding, rectal bleeding, melena, hematochezia, hematuria, sexual activity, or STIs. She denies anxiety or depression.

Relevant History

The patient had recurrent tonsillitis when she was younger, which resolved with tonsillectomy at age 8, acute appendicitis at age 12, and a fracture of left foot 4 months ago. Her mother has IBS and T1DM, and her father and two brothers have no health conditions. She has a maternal aunt with celiac sprue and a maternal grandmother diagnosed with celiac sprue, T1DM, and thyroid disease.

Allergies

No known drug allergies; no known food allergies.

Medications

None.

Physical Examination

- *Vitals:* T 37°C (98.6°F), P 74, R 14, BP 100/68, HT 160.02 cm (63 in.), WT 49.90 kg (110 lb), BMI 19.5.
- *General:* Patient appears in no acute distress, well developed, pale in appearance.
- *Psychiatric:* Normal mood and affect.
- *Skin, Hair, and Nails:* Papulovesicular rash on extensor surface with mild excoriations located on BL lower legs. Normal skin turgor. No abnormal findings with hair or nails.
- *Eyes:* Conjunctivae are pale.

- *ENT/Mouth:* TM appear pearly gray with normal landmarks; nose with boggy turbinates and clear rhinorrhea; oral mucosa is moist; no ulcerations, no oropharyngeal erythema; tonsils are absent; several dental caries in upper and lower molars.
- *Lungs:* CTAs bilaterally.
- *Heart:* RRR, with no murmurs, gallops, or rubs.
- *Abdomen:* Soft, mildly distended with no masses, guarding, or rigidity. No hepatosplenomegaly. Negative Murphy sign, McBurney point, and psoas and obturator tests.
- *Musculoskeletal:* No joint swelling or tenderness; ROM of all joints are normal.
- *Genital/Rectal:* No perianal skin tags, fistulas, or abscess. No masses or retained stool on digital rectal exam. Negative occult fecal blood testing.

Clinical Discussion Questions

1. What is the differential diagnosis?

____

____

____

____

2. What is the most likely diagnosis? Why?

____

____

____

____

3. Demonstrate your understanding about the pathophysiology of the most likely diagnosis.

____

____

____

____

4. Should tests/imaging studies be ordered? Which ones? Why? Think about tests/imaging beyond the primary care setting as well.

____

____

____

____

5. What are the next appropriate steps in management?

6. Review reliable, recent references and demonstrate an understanding of the diagnostic approach, treatment, and follow-up recommendations for this diagnosis. Include the name of the source(s).

7. What are the pertinent ICD-10 and CPT (E/M) codes for this visit? Provide a short rationale.

8. What is the appropriate patient education topic for this case?

9. If not managed appropriately, what is/are the medical/legal concern(s) that may arise?

10. Think about interprofessional collaboration for this case. Provide a list of specialties or other disciplines and indicate what contribution these professionals might make to managing the patient.

BEDSIDE MANNER QUESTION

11. What would your communication style/approach be with this patient and her mother?

Answers available at courseconnect.springerpub.com.

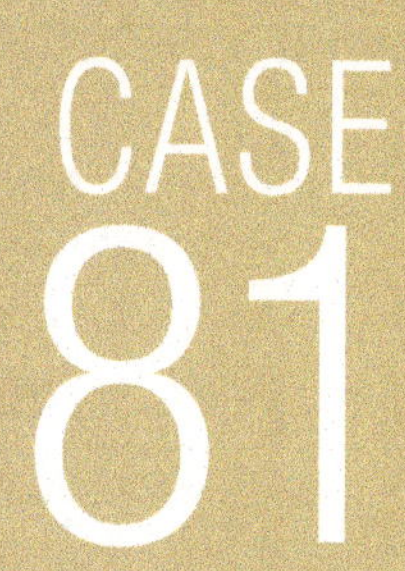

REFUSAL TO EAT OR DRINK, PEDIATRIC MALE

Chief Complaint

"Refusal to eat or drink."

History of Present Illness

A mother brings her 5-year-old son to his PCP for evaluation of a 2-day refusal to eat and drink. The mother reports the child has been extremely fussy; he has not been sleeping well, wakes up crying, and is hard to console. The mother states the child was hot to touch but she was unable to measure his temperature because she does not have a thermometer. She has been giving him children's acetaminophen and diphenhydramine to help with fussiness and sleep. The mother denies vomiting or diarrhea by the child. She adds he was well and active 2 days ago. The mother denies sick contact with his other sibling but did note that there are other children at day care with similar symptoms.

Review of Systems

The patient's ROS is positive for fever, excessive irritability, refusal to eat or drink, and fatigue. His ROS is negative for vomiting, diarrhea, abdominal pain, headache, difficulty talking, runny nose, or persistent cough.

Relevant History

The child's medical history is significant for a full-term birth at 39 weeks without pregnancy complications. His immunizations are up to date. He has no history of hospitalizations and no chronic medical conditions. He has met all developmental milestones and growth trajectories without concern. He lives with his parents, attends pre-K day care full-time, and eats a balanced diet. His mother and father are healthy. They have no chronic medical conditions.

Allergies

No known drug, food, or environmental allergies.

Medications

None.

Physical Examination

- *Vitals:* T 38.4°C (101.2°F), P 118, R 20, BP 110/80, HT 109.2 (43 in.), WT 19.1 kg (42 lb), BMI 16.
- *General:* Alert, fussy and irritable, seems fatigued.
- *Skin, Hair, and Nails:* No abnormal findings. No rash.
- *Head:* Normocephalic and atraumatic.
- *ENT/Mouth:* Oropharyngeal and tonsillar area with moderate beefy red erythema with white exudates; no stridor noted; no uvular deviation noted; patient is tolerating oral secretions; no tripod position noted. Surface of the oral mucosa and tongue without abnormal findings.

- *Neck:* Neck is soft, supple, with adequate ROM; no nuchal rigidity noted; tender adenopathy in anterior and posterior cervical chain present.
- *Lungs:* CTA bilaterally with equal and symmetrical respiratory excursion.
- *Heart:* RRR; no murmur or gallops noted.
- *Abdomen:* Soft, not distended, appears nontender.
- *Neurologic:* CN II to XII are grossly intact; no problem with gait or balance noted.

CLINICAL DISCUSSION QUESTIONS

1. What is the differential diagnosis?

2. What is the most likely diagnosis? Why?

3. Demonstrate your understanding about the pathophysiology of the most likely diagnosis.

4. Should tests/imaging studies be ordered? Which ones? Why? Think about tests/imaging beyond the primary care setting as well.

5. What are the next appropriate steps in management?

6. What is the most common cause of and treatment for this diagnosis in children, and what are the risks associated with a missed diagnosis? Provide references for your response.

7. What are the pertinent ICD-10 and CPT (E/M) codes for this visit? Provide a short rationale.

8. What is the appropriate parent education topic for this case?

9. If not managed appropriately, what is/are the medical/legal concern(s) that may arise?

10. Think about interprofessional collaboration for this case. Provide a list of specialties or other disciplines and indicate what contribution these professionals might make to managing the patient.

Bedside Manner Question

11. What would your communication style/approach be with this parent?

___

___

___

___

Answers available at courseconnect.springerpub.com.

CASE 82

BACK PAIN AND POOR POSTURE, PEDIATRIC FEMALE

Chief Complaint

"Back pain and poor posture."

History of Present Illness

A 9-year-old girl is brought to the office by her parents to discuss her poor posture and lingering back pain. They constantly remind her to sit up straight. Their daughter states she tries to sit straight and is doing the best she can. She admits to lingering mid-back pain. The pain is a 4/10, is localized to mid-thoracic area bilaterally, does not migrate, and is described as a consistent ache, not stabbing or pulsatile. The patient takes ibuprofen 200 mg Q6h sometimes but usually tries to just ignore her pain. She is not involved in any sports but plays violin and piano. She is active with friends and has not noted any change or limitation in interactions with them. She denies pain in her shoulders or legs. No muscle weakness in her extremities has been noted by her or her parents. They state this has been going on for a while and think they noted the problem the most over the past 6 to 9 months.

Review of Systems

The ROS was unremarkable. The girl has mid-thoracic BL 4/10 pain as described. The ROS was negative for cough, SOB, chest pain, fatigue, abdominal pain, vomiting, diarrhea, dysuria, fever, muscle weakness, or dizziness.

Relevant History

The patient is fully vaccinated and has had no recent travel; she has no history of prior surgeries or trauma and no chronic health concerns. Her parents recall she reached developmental milestones on time. She has not been to a pediatrician since her kindergarten checkup because her parents' insurance has a high deductible. The child lives with her parents in a house built about 10 years ago. Her parents deny any significant family history of illness.

Allergies

No known food or drug allergies.

Medications

Ibuprofen 200 mg Q6h PRN for pain.

Physical Examination

- *Vitals:* T 37°C (98.6°F); P 80; R 17; BP 116/72; WT 41.27 kg (91 lb), 90th to 95th percentile; HT 147.32 cm (58 in.), 95th to 100th percentile; BMI 19.
- *General:* Alert and in no distress.
- *Skin, Hair, and Nails:* Warm, dry, with no rashes noted. Capillary refill brisk. No abnormal findings with hair or nails.
- *Head:* Normocephalic and atraumatic.
- *Neck:* Supple with no adenopathy.
- *Chest:* The sternum is normal, with no pectus carinatum or excavatum noted.

- *Lungs:* CTA throughout all fields. Aeration is symmetric.
- *Heart:* RRR, with no murmur, gallop, or rub.
- *Abdomen:* Soft, nontender, nondistended with no masses noted. BS equal throughout.
- *Genital/ Rectal:* Tanner stage 1. Rectal exam deferred.
- *Musculoskeletal:* Obvious shoulder height discrepancy with right shoulder elevated. Right scapula is mildly elevated compared to the left. A forward bend test shows noticeable prominence to the right thoracic and ribs in the mid-thoracic range. There is also prominence to the paraspinal muscles of the left lumbar spine. A scoliometer is utilized and shows a 9° angle of rotation over the mid-thoracic spine and 7° angle of rotation over the lumbar spine.
- *Neurologic:* CN II to XII intact. DTR symmetric in the upper and lower extremities at 2/4, and muscle strength symmetric in the upper and lower extremities at 5/5.

Clinical Discussion Questions

1. What is the differential diagnosis?

___

___

___

___

2. What is the most likely diagnosis? Why?

___

___

___

___

3. Demonstrate your understanding about the pathophysiology of the most likely diagnosis.

___

___

___

___

4. Should tests/imaging studies be ordered? Which ones? Why? Think about tests/imaging beyond the primary care setting as well.

___

___

___

___

5. What are the next appropriate steps in management?

6. Discuss screening and treatment recommendations for the diagnosis. Additionally, what role do CM play in the diagnosis? Include references to support your response.

7. What are the pertinent ICD-10 and CPT (E/M) codes for this visit? Provide a short rationale.

8. What is the appropriate patient education topic for this case?

9. If not managed appropriately, what is/are the medical/legal concern(s) that may arise?

10. Think about interprofessional collaboration for this case. Provide a list of specialties or other disciplines and indicate what contribution these professionals might make to managing the patient.

Bedside Manner Questions

11. How would you communicate your likely diagnosis to the patient and her parents?

12. If the patient and family show distress at what you communicate, how would you provide support?

Answers available at courseconnect.springerpub.com.

ITCHY BUMPS, PEDIATRIC FEMALE

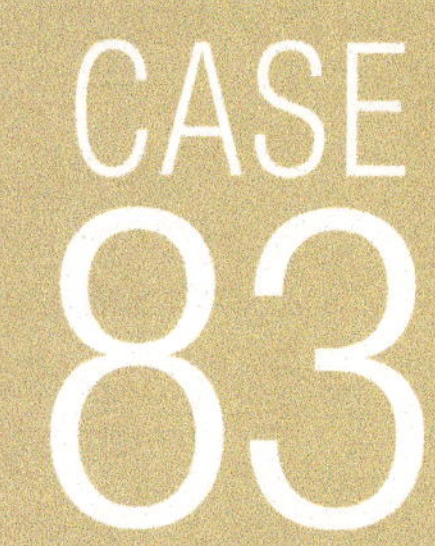

Chief Complaint

"Itchy bumps."

History of Present Illness

A mother brings her 9-year-old daughter to her PCP for evaluation of an itchy, bumpy rash that comes and goes but resolves within a few hours. This has been going on for 1 month. The last episode of rash was 1 day ago and lasted all day—keeping the child and parent up at night. The rash was accompanied by a swelling of the girl's eyelids. The mother administered diphenhydramine at night, which helped a little. Today, the eye swelling has resolved and the rash is slightly better. The mother was able to take some pictures of the initial rash with her phone. The rash in the pictures shows raised bumps and patches, round or oval across the body, especially on the abdomen, thigh, and back. The patient remembers having a few itchy bumps here and there in the past but thought they were mosquito bites. The patient and mother cannot recall a correlation between rash and possible triggers such as food, contact, or other stressors such as heat, cold, or medications such as NSAIDs. The mother is extremely concerned as she has tried to find answers online and worried her child may have leukemia or another type of cancer. The mother is unaware of her daughter having any food allergies.

Review of Systems

The patient's ROS is positive for diffuse rash, pruritus, and upper eyelid swelling. Her ROS is negative for unexplained fever, adenopathy, recent unintentional weight loss, fatigue, headache, joint pain or swelling, wheezing, flushing, palpitation, abdominal pain, skin ulceration, wheezing, SOB, and swelling of throat or tongue. She has no history of thyroid dysfunction, vasculitis, or autoimmune-related health problems.

Relevant History

The patient has a history of seasonal allergies to pollen and takes loratadine 10 mg QD during spring and early summer. She is up to date on her immunizations. There is no significant contributory history from her family.

Allergies

No known drug allergies; no known food allergies.

Medications

Loratadine 10 mg PO QD PRN for seasonal allergies.

Physical Examination

- *Vitals:* T 37°C (98.6°F), P 80, R 18, BP 110/72, WT 36.29 kg (80 lb), HT 142.24 cm (56 in.), BMI 18.
- *General:* A&O, playful, and interactive.
- *Psychiatry:* Normal affect, good eye contact, answers general questions appropriately.
- *Skin, Hair, and Nails:* No lesions or scales in hairline noted. Diffuse raised erythematous and edematous papules and plaques ranging from 0.2 cm to 1 cm present on neck, abdomen,

thigh, legs, arm, hands, feet, buttocks, and back. Plantar and palmer surfaces are spared. Lesions are blanchable. No ulceration or target lesion noted. No jaundice noted. Skin has a normal turgor. No abnormal findings with hair or nails.

- *Eyes:* Both eyes with clear sclera and conjunctiva; ophthalmoscope exam shows no sign of hemorrhage.
- *ENT/Mouth:* Both TM clear with cone of light visible; oropharyngeal mucosa without redness or exudate. No swelling of eyelids, lips, or tongue.
- *Neck:* Nontender, no adenopathy noted.
- *Lungs:* No wheezing, rales, or rhonchi.
- *Heart:* RRR, no murmur noted.
- *Peripheral Vascular:* Good peripheral perfusion present.

Clinical Discussion Questions

1. What is the differential diagnosis?

____

____

____

____

2. What is the most likely diagnosis? Why?

____

____

____

____

3. Demonstrate your understanding about the pathophysiology of the most likely diagnosis.

____

____

____

____

4. Should tests/imaging studies be ordered? Which ones? Why? Think about tests/imaging beyond the primary care setting as well.

____

____

____

____

5. What are the next appropriate steps in management?

6. What is the diagnostic approach and prognosis for this diagnosis? Provide references for your response.

7. What are the pertinent ICD-10 and CPT (E/M) codes for this visit? Provide a short rationale.

8. What is the appropriate patient education topic for this case?

9. If not managed appropriately, what is/are the medical/legal concern(s) that may arise?

10. Think about interprofessional collaboration for this case. Provide a list of specialties or other disciplines and indicate what contribution these professionals might make to managing the patient.

Bedside Manner Question

11. What would your communication style/approach be with this parent/patient?

Answers available at courseconnect.springerpub.com.

NUMBNESS IN HANDS AND LEGS, GERIATRIC MALE

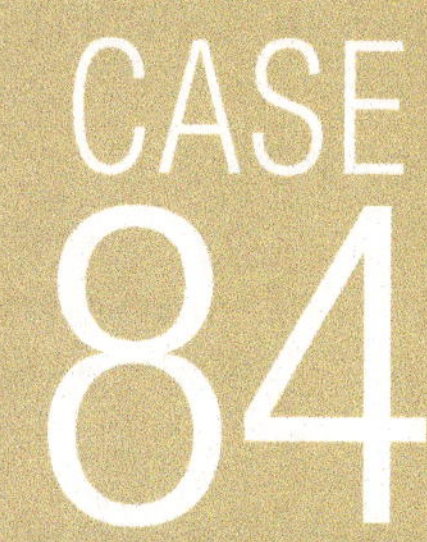

Chief Complaint

"Numbness in hands and legs."

History of Present Illness

A 65-year-old man presents to his PCP with an initial complaint of insidious onset of hand and leg numbness and weakness. He describes tingling and weakness over the last 3 days. He has numbness in a glove-like pattern to both hands and distal forearms as well as numbness and weakness to his lower extremities. He admits to dropping items and cannot shake off the tingling and sense of imbalance because of the numbness in his feet. He says he has difficulty getting out of his recliner and describes progressive, worsening numbness and weakness just over the last day. He also admits to precedent pain to extremities prior to onset of numbness. He has pain in his upper and lower limbs that he describes as a dull, nonradiating ache with severity five to six of 10 at its worst. The patient states the discomfort has interfered with his sleep, contributing to his fatigue. He has a history of a MVA 15 years ago, when his car was rear-ended, and he sustained a lower back and whiplash injury. He states after a year of physical therapy, his painful condition resolved and he was able to resume work. The patient states, "My neck and back pain had been fine for years until 5 days ago." He has no prior surgeries to back or upper extremities. He admits to recent illness, about 3 weeks ago, which he describes as bad "food poisoning" and experienced diarrhea for 5 days with malaise, fatigue, and weight loss of 10 lb. He was seen by urgent care, closer to home, and was reassured that he had an occurrence of viral gastroenteritis. Since then, he has been fatigued with loss of appetite and been unable to regain his lost weight. He states, "It hit me hard and sapped the energy out of me." He is here today with his wife.

Review of Systems

The ROS is positive for decreased appetite; fatigue; nausea; insomnia; occasional dizziness; and some mild blurring of vision and imbalance problems related to numbness, weakness, and tingling of feet. He denies fever, chills, nausea, vomiting, worsening of chronic headaches, tinnitus, diplopia, dysphagia, SOB, dyspnea on exertion, orthopnea, chest pain, palpitations, paroxysmal nocturnal dyspnea, abdominal pain, current diarrhea, or constipation. The patient has good bowel and bladder control.

Relevant History

The patient's medical history is significant for well-controlled HTN and hyperlipidemia. He had musculoskeletal neck and back pain for a year after a car accident and was treated conservatively to resolution.

The patient is married with two children and works for the postal service. Active prior to the recent illness, he enjoyed hiking and biking at least once a week with his wife. He does not smoke and has one glass of wine with dinner each evening. He has no history of recreational drug use. He had the usual childhood illnesses. His family history is noncontributory except for a mother with lupus.

Allergies

No known drug allergies; no known food allergies.

MEDICATIONS

- Lisinopril 20 mg PO QD.
- Atorvastatin 20 mg PO QHS.
- Daily multivitamin.

PHYSICAL EXAMINATION

- *Vitals:* T 37°C (98.6°F), P 98, R 14, BP 140/90, WT 82.5 kg (182 lb), HT 175 cm (69 in.), BMI 27.
- *General:* The patient is in no apparent distress and is ambulatory without an assistive device. He has a slightly ataxic gait and holds onto hallway rails.
- *Psychiatric:* A&O and conversant individual. Good historian. Good judgment and insight.
- *Skin, Hair, and Nails:* No lesions, rashes. Hair and nails unremarkable. Hair present to lower extremities and dorsum feet, with even distribution bilaterally.
- *Head:* Normocephalic. Atraumatic.
- *Eyes:* PERRLA. EOMI.
- *ENT/Mouth:* Oral mucosa with good dentition. Gross hearing intact. BL TM intact and not inflamed.
- *Neck:* FROM. Trachea midline. No adenopathy.
- *Chest:* Symmetrical. No axillary adenopathy.
- *Lungs:* BL clear lung fields with good air movement.
- *Heart:* RRR, without murmur or gallop.
- *Abdomen:* Abdomen soft, nontender, BS intact in all quadrants. No discernible organomegaly.
- *Genital/Rectal:* No anal lesions. Good sphincter tone. Normal male genitalia.
- *Musculoskeletal:* Mild BL paraspinous tenderness with deep palpation to base of neck extending to the mid-interscapular areas and laterally to posterior shoulders. No nuchal rigidity. No scapular winging. Active FROM to neck and shoulder with end range discomfort. BL hands warm and dry. Allen test negative. Grasp equal but weak symmetrically. No intrinsic muscle wasting noted. Tinel sign noted with pain elicited to forearm. Phalen sign negative. Hypoesthesia both dorsal and volar aspects of hand extending to wrist in glove-like pattern.
- Lower lumbosacral spine without tenderness. Straight leg raises negative bilaterally. Lhermitte sign negative. Lower extremities with active FROM. Motor 4/5 to knees and 4/5 ankles. Hypoesthesia to BL feet and ankles extending to distal calf in glove-like pattern with poor discrimination testing to sharp and dull.
- *Neurologic:* CN II to XII grossly intact. No facial paresis noted. Deep tendon reflexes: triceps: 1+; brachioradialis/biceps: absent; radial: absent; patellar: 1+; ankle: absent with reinforcement.
- *Vascular:* Peripheral pulses (dorsalis pedis, posterior tibial, radial and ulnar) all 2+ bilaterally. Normal hair growth in lower and upper extremities with quick capillary refill bilateral toes and fingers.

CLINICAL DISCUSSION QUESTIONS

1. What is the differential diagnosis?

____

____

____

____

2. What is the most likely diagnosis? Why?

3. Demonstrate your understanding about the pathophysiology of the most likely diagnosis.

4. Should tests/imaging studies be ordered? Which ones? Why? Think about tests/imaging beyond the primary care setting as well.

5. What are the next appropriate steps in management?

6. What are the triggers, associated microorganisms, critical predictors, and complications of the disease? Provide references for your response.

7. What are the pertinent ICD-10 and CPT (E/M) codes for this visit? Provide a short rationale.

8. What is the appropriate patient education topic for this case?

9. If not managed appropriately, what is/are the medical/legal concern(s) that may arise?

10. Think about interprofessional collaboration for this case. Provide a list of specialties or other disciplines and indicate what contribution these professionals might make to managing the patient.

BEDSIDE MANNER QUESTIONS

11. What would your communication style/approach be with this patient and his wife?

12. If a patient and his wife are distressed by the diagnosis, what might offer support?

Answers available at courseconnect.springerpub.com.

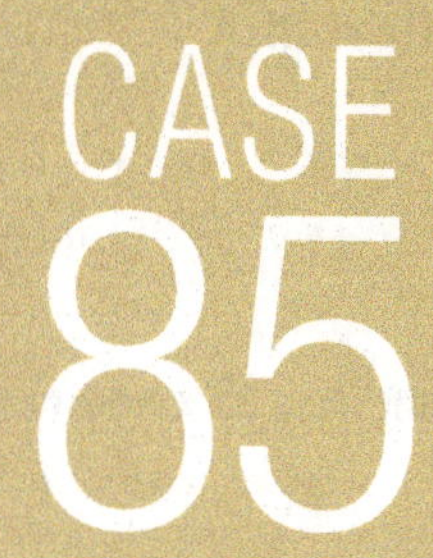

PAINFUL RASH, GERIATRIC MALE

CASE 85

Chief Complaint

"Painful rash."

History of Present Illness

A 68-year-old man presents to his PCP with a 1-week history of thoracic pain. He describes the pain as slow onset of symptoms on the right side of his thoracic spine radiating to his anterior trunk. The pain has progressively worsened and he describes it as sharp and burning. He states the discomfort started a week ago as an ache after returning home from work. He suspected a strained muscle and treated with warm packs and OTC ibuprofen. In the subsequent days, his pain became worse and he was concerned he had irreversibly injured his back. He denies any associated paresthesia or recent weight loss.

About 2 days ago, he noticed a mildly pruritic rash to his abdomen and he was not sure if this was related to his pain. He states, "It even hurts to breathe now," noting that positional changes make the pain worse. He states it is very tender to lay on his right side.

He is a fieldworker; he drives heavy equipment and supervises other workers. He is concerned he injured his back getting in or out of equipment, which occurs frequently during a normal workday.

Review of Systems

The ROS is positive for difficulty sleeping related to right upper abdominal pain, fatigue, mild dyspepsia, decreased appetite, and mild dyspnea on exertion related to pain. The ROS is negative for fever, chills, cough, vomiting, sick contacts, melena, hematochezia, liver disease, HIV, headache, dizziness, blurred vision, recent travel requiring prolonged sitting, paroxysmal nocturnal dyspnea, lower extremity, palpitations, paresthesia, or muscle weakness.

Relevant History

The patient's medical history is significant for well-controlled T2DM, HTN, hyperlipidemia, and obesity. His surgical history is significant for cholecystectomy (age 48), colonoscopy, and upper endoscopy (age 65) revealing mild gastritis. He admits to usual childhood illnesses. Social history is significant for one to two beers after work daily. The patient quit smoking cigarettes at age 48 and denies recreational drug use. He is heterosexual with no history of sexually transmitted infections and enjoys a monogamous relationship with his wife. He has three grown children, nine grandchildren, and one great-grandson. He resides in a single-story home with his wife. He is the primary wage earner. He states a granddaughter is reliant on him for college funding. His family history is unknown.

Allergies

No known drug allergies; no known food allergies.

Medications

- Metformin 1,000 mg PO BID.
- Glargine insulin 15 units SQ QD.
- Atorvastatin 20 mg QD.
- Lisinopril 20 mg PO QD.

- Aspirin 81 mg PO QD.
- Fish oil (omega 3) 1,000 mg PO QD.

PHYSICAL EXAMINATION

- *Vitals:* T 37°C (98.6°F), P 88, R 14, BP 138/82, WT 85 kg (188 lb), HT 170 cm (67 in.), BMI 29.
- *General:* Spanish-speaking male. Grimacing and appears in pain with guarded movements.
- *Psychiatric:* Good historian with linear thought processes.
- *Skin, Hair, and Nails:* Right sub xiphoid area with 1- to 2- cm papular vesicular rash on background of hyperemia in clusters, extending laterally to midclavicular line in dermatomal pattern. Few dispersed vesicles noted. No lymphadenopathy to axilla. No other lesions or rashes noted. Hair and nails unremarkable. Hair present to lower extremities and dorsum feet, with even distribution bilaterally.
- *Head:* Normocephalic, atraumatic.
- *Eyes:* PERRLA, EOMI.
- *ENT/Mouth:* Dentition in good repair. Gross hearing intact. BL TMs patent.
- *Neck:* FROM, trachea midline, no adenopathy.
- *Chest:* Symmetrical, no axillary adenopathy.
- *Lungs:* CTA bilaterally. Good air movement discernible.
- *Heart:* RRR, without murmur/gallop.
- *Back:* No spinous tenderness. Right back tender to touch at approximately T7; inferior angle of scapula level. FROM neck with flexion, extension, lateral and rotational movements. FROM left and right shoulder without scapular winging.
- *Abdomen:* Protuberant. Moderate tenderness right upper quadrant and epigastric area to light touch. No peritoneal signs. No ascites. Murphy sign negative. Negative rebound.
- *Neurologic:* CN II to XII intact. Hyperesthesia right T7 to T8 dermatomes; otherwise normal gross motor sensation in upper and lower extremities.

CLINICAL DISCUSSION QUESTIONS

1. What is the differential diagnosis?

____

____

____

____

2. What is the most likely diagnosis? Why?

____

____

____

____

3. Demonstrate your understanding about the pathophysiology of the most likely diagnosis.

4. Should tests/imaging studies be ordered? Which ones? Why? Think about tests/imaging beyond the primary care setting as well.

5. What are the next appropriate steps in management?

6. Review reliable articles and investigate the prevalence, treatment options, associated symptom(s), and recurrence of the diagnosis. Include the name of the references.

7. What are the pertinent ICD-10 and CPT (E/M) codes for this visit? Provide a short rationale.

8. What is the appropriate patient education topic for this case?

9. If not managed appropriately, what is/are the medical/legal concern(s) that may arise?

10. Think about interprofessional collaboration for this case. Provide a list of specialties or other disciplines and indicate what contribution these professionals might make to managing the patient.

BEDSIDE MANNER QUESTION

11. What would your communication style/approach be with this patient?

Answers available at courseconnect.springerpub.com.

SPEECH DIFFICULTIES, GERIATRIC MALE

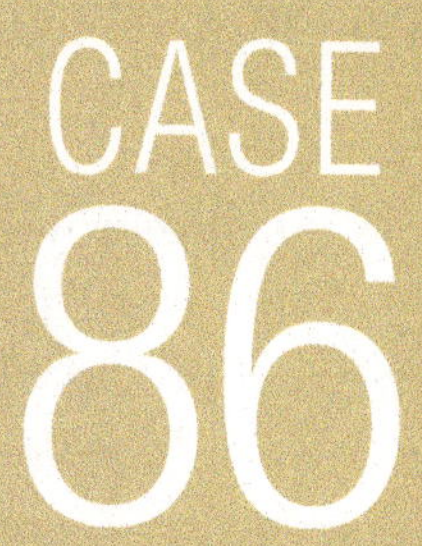

CHIEF COMPLAINT

"Speech difficulties."

HISTORY OF PRESENT ILLNESS

A 74-year-old man, accompanied by his son, presents for evaluation of speech changes over the past 6 months. The patient denies significant change in voice, but his son provides history that his father's voice has grown softer, speech is now slowly produced, and it is difficult to understand him at times. This has made communication over the phone particularly challenging. The patient's son lives out of state, so he had not seen his father in person for about 8 months and they rely on phone communication. The patient's son states he was a bit surprised upon seeing his dad because he noted not only the voice and speech pattern changes but also a tremor in his right hand. The patient denies experiencing any falls in the last year.

REVIEW OF SYSTEMS

The ROS is positive for skin dryness, increasingly vivid dreams, and tremor in the right hand. The patient's ROS is negative for anxiety, depression, weight loss, or fatigue. No recent or other trauma stated. He is negative for head injuries recently or in the past. No numbness, tingling, or paresthesia in the hand(s) noted.

MEDICAL HISTORY

The patient denies use of prescription medications or chronic medical conditions. He takes a men's daily multivitamin but no other supplements. His social history includes one 3-ounce serving of whiskey each night before bed. Alcohol does not seem to affect the tremor. He was a tobacco smoker, 1 pack per day for 15 years, but quit 25 years ago. He denies illicit drug use now or in the past. He denies exposure to neurotoxins or other chemicals. His family history includes mother, deceased, at age 94, natural causes; father, deceased, at 56, MVA; a younger sister, 68, with hyperthyroid and depression, which are managed; one adult son, an adult daughter, and three granddaughters, all healthy. He was widowed 3 years ago. He denies any family history of tremor.

ALLERGIES

Penicillin (hives); no known food allergies.

MEDICATIONS

Men's daily multivitamin, generic.

PHYSICAL EXAMINATION

- *Vitals:* T 37°C (98.6°F), P 78, R 22, BP 110/78, HT 182.88 cm (72 in.), WT 80.28 kg (177 lb); BMI 24.
- *General:* Well nourished, good hygiene, no acute distress, decreased spontaneous facial expressions.
- *Psychiatric:* Able to follow commands, cooperative with physical exam, slow to answer history questions.

- *Skin, Hair, and Nails:* Seborrheic dermatitis present around the nasal labial folds and eyebrows.
- *ENT/Mouth:* Voice quality poor (low volume); speech lacks spontaneity and fluidity when produced; EOMI in six cardinal positions of gaze.
- *Musculoskeletal:* 5/5 strength in BL UE and BLE; no atrophy of musculature or reduced ROM.
- *Neurologic:* DTRs 2+ equal and symmetrical in BL UE and BLE; positive for glabellar reflex; no increased tone through passive motion in left UE or BLE; right UE exhibits cogwheeling at the wrist and elbow that worsens with distraction; supination-pronation tremor noted at rest in the right hand; slight jaw tremor noted; gait/balance assessment: patient needed three attempts to rise from the chair using hands, positive retropulsion test, shuffling gait present with reduced stride length; reduced arm swing in the right arm on ambulation; negative Romberg sensation intact to light and sharp touch on plantar surfaces of feet bilaterally; writing assessment: handwriting is small and illegible, impaired ability to copy a spiral (patient's rendition appears smaller with less fluid lines compared to provider's example); rapid alternating movements impaired in the right upper extremity; Mini-Mental State Exam score = 26/30.

Clinical Discussion Questions

1. What is the differential diagnosis?

2. What is the most likely diagnosis? Why?

3. Demonstrate your understanding about pathophysiology of the most likely diagnosis.

4. Should tests/imaging studies be ordered? Which ones? Why? Think about tests/imaging beyond the primary care setting as well.

5. What are the next appropriate steps in management?

6. What are the clinical presentations, diagnostic criteria, and treatment approaches for this diagnosis? Provide references for your response.

7. What are the pertinent ICD-10 and CPT (E/M) codes for this visit? Provide a short rationale.

8. What is the appropriate patient education topic for this case?

9. If not managed appropriately, what is/are the medical/legal concern(s) that may arise?

10. Think about interprofessional collaboration for this case. Provide a list of specialties or other disciplines and indicate what contribution these professionals might make to managing the patient.

Bedside Manner Questions

11. What would your communication style/approach be with this patient and his son?

12. If a patient and his son are distressed by the diagnosis, what might offer support?

Answers available at courseconnect.springerpub.com.

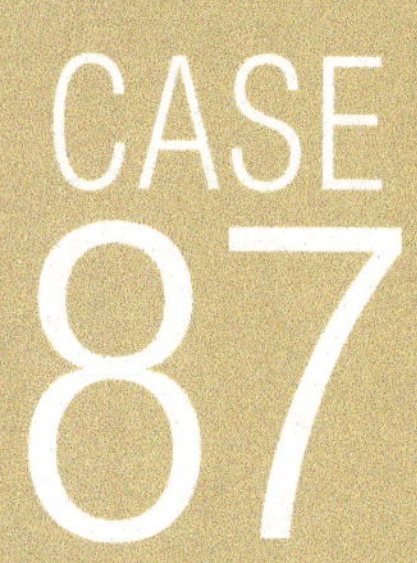

FEVER AND BACK PAIN, GERIATRIC FEMALE

Chief Complaint

"Fever and back pain."

History of Present Illness

A 78-year-old woman presents to her regular PCP with a 2-day history of fatigue, malaise, and fever. She awoke this morning with a dull ache in her right mid-back and some nausea. She came to the office because she is concerned about the pain and her worsening symptoms. She has been resting and taking acetaminophen (650 mg every 4 to 6 hours), which has helped with the fever and aches, but her symptoms return as the drug wears off. She is unsure of how high her fever has gotten. She states the pain is a 3 or 4 out of 10, but the fatigue, malaise, and nausea have kept her from her daily activities and caused her to stay in bed most of yesterday and today. She believes she might have "the flu" though she received the vaccine 3 weeks ago. She is most concerned because she lives alone and is afraid of becoming seriously ill and having no way to call for help. She denies ever smoking and drinks a glass of wine only once or twice a month. Her husband of many years died 8 years ago of prostate cancer and she lives independently in an apartment. One of her three children lives a few miles away and visits frequently. She is not currently sexually active.

She denies chills, night sweats, rhinorrhea, cough, SOB, dyspnea, chest pains, palpitations, vomiting, diarrhea, or constipation. She admits to increased urinary frequency and urgency but denies pain with urination. She denies sick contacts or changes to her dietary routine.

Review of Systems

The patient's ROS is positive for occasional knee pain. Her ROS is negative for weakness, weight loss, focal pain except in the right flank, difficulty with memory or concentration, recent illness, or injury.

Relevant History

The patient's history is significant for HTN and osteoporosis. She has a family history of CAD. Her daughter lives nearby and is available to stay with her if needed.

Allergies

No medication, environmental, or food allergies.

Medications

- Lisinopril/hydrochlorothiazide 10/12.5 mg QD.
- Alendronate 70 mg weekly.
- OTC 1,000 mg calcium citrate with 600 IU vitamin D3 QD.

Physical Examination

- *Vitals:* T 38.8°C (101.8°F), P 96, R 14, BP 106/68, WT 56.7 kg (125 lb), HT 172.72 cm (68 in.), BMI 20.2.
- *General:* Ill and uncomfortable appearing, but nontoxic and without acute distress.
- *Psychiatric:* A&O×3; coherent conversation.
- *Skin, Hair, and Nails:* Skin pale and slightly flushed, no rash or lesion. Nails are smooth without hemorrhage.

- *Eye:* Eyes without retinal lesions.
- *ENT/Mouth:* Oral mucosa moist without lesions.
- *Chest:* Symmetric excursion with no accessory muscle use.
- *Breasts:* No mass or lesion bilaterally.
- *Lungs:* Resonant with vesicular breath sounds all fields; no wheezes, rales, or rhonchi.
- *Heart:* Quiet precordium; RSR; no murmur, rub, or gallop.
- *Abdomen:* Flat, NABS all quadrants, no mass. There is mild right costovertebral angle tenderness and mild suprapubic discomfort but no tenderness.
- *Genital/Rectal:* Vaginal and introital mucosa show atrophy. The uterus is small and smooth. No mass or lesion detected in the adnexa or cul-de-sac.
- *Musculoskeletal:* No point tenderness detected on the vertebral processes.

Clinical Discussion Questions

1. What is the differential diagnosis?

2. What is the most likely diagnosis? Why?

3. Demonstrate your understanding about pathophysiology of the most likely diagnosis.

4. Should tests/imaging studies be ordered? Which ones? Why? Think about tests/imaging beyond the primary care setting as well.

5. What are the next appropriate steps in management?

6. Review a recent and credible research article about the key factors (causes, risks, diagnostic testing, and treatment selection) of this diagnosis. Provide references for your response.

7. What are the pertinent ICD-10 and CPT (E/M) codes for this visit? Provide a short rationale.

8. What is the appropriate patient education topic for this case?

9. If not managed appropriately, what is/are the medical/legal concern(s) that may arise?

10. Think about interprofessional collaboration for this case. Provide a list of specialties or other disciplines and indicate what contribution these professionals might make to managing the patient.

BEDSIDE MANNER QUESTION

11. What would your communication style/approach be with this patient?

____

____

____

____

Answers available at courseconnect.springerpub.com.

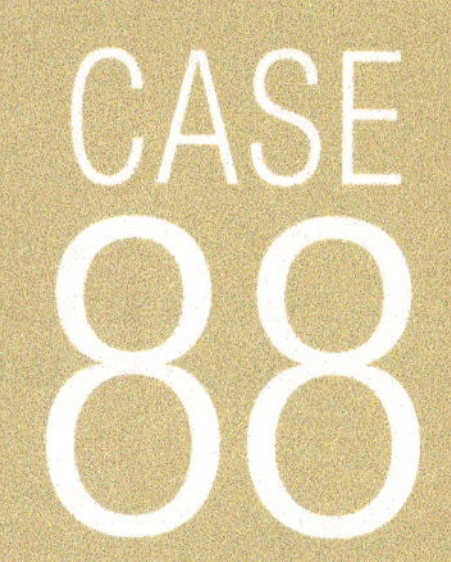

MALAISE AND RIGHT-SIDE PAIN, GERIATRIC MALE

Chief Complaint

"General malaise, right-side pain."

History of Present Illness

A 65-year-old avid bicyclist with HTN and hyperlipidemia is brought in by his wife, stating he is feeling "not myself" today. He could not make his daily 20-mile bike ride this morning, which he has not missed in 10 years, due to sharp right-sided "rib pain" that radiates to his right axilla and shoulder. The pain, ranging from one to nine out of 10 in severity, began 2 days ago, several minutes after returning from his bike ride. He states it "feels like the muscles between the ribs and assumes he "pulled something" in his chest. He also experienced identical chest pain on the left side 1 day prior, shortly after biking, which resolved completely after taking a muscle relaxant. Last night, he developed a fever of 38.3°C (101° F), night sweats, and the inability to take a deep breath or lie flat without severe "rib pain"—despite taking the muscle relaxant, he had to sleep sitting up. The patient's wife confirms he has been very compliant with taking his prescribed daily medications; however, the patient admits that 3 months ago, he stopped taking the daily baby aspirin prescribed by his cardiologist because he read a news report that aspirin "isn't recommended anymore."

Regarding his recent health, the patient went to urgent care a week ago for left calf pain and swelling which began 5 days prior, while flying home to Los Angeles from a 3-day trip to New York. He states the urgent care doctor measured his left calf as 1 cm greater than the right but told him it "didn't look swollen," so no further tests were recommended. He continued to bike daily since then, and today, his leg pain is better; however, the swelling has worsened, moving into his left ankle and foot.

The patient states he had a "24-hour flu" while in New York, described as diffuse abdominal pain, myalgias, fatigue, and anorexia, without any associated fever, cough, nausea, vomiting or diarrhea. Symptoms self-resolved, and no one else had similar symptoms. He has had 4 similar episodes in the last 5 years, always when flying, but he has never sought care, as they quickly resolved.

Review of Systems

The patient's ROS is positive for nonpruritic red rash over left lower leg x 1 week. His ROS is negative for weight loss, fatigue, cough, hemoptysis, or SOB. He has no palpitations, dizziness, or syncope. The patient has no current abdominal pain and no nausea/vomiting. He denies change in bowel movements, melena, or hematochezia. No weakness, paresthesia, or dysarthria. No anxiety or depression.

Relevant History

The patient has essential HTN, hyperlipidemia, impaired fasting glucose, and an abnormal EKG with first-degree AV block; last stress test and echocardiograms were normal 1 year ago. His conditions are well controlled on lisinopril 20 mg QD and atorvastatin 40 mg QD, along with vigorous exercise and a low-carbohydrate diet. He takes cyclobenzaprine 10 mg occasionally PRN for flares of chronic lumbar strain; states he "never gets sick."

The patient underwent left testicular torsion surgery in 1974 and has no history of blood transfusion. He had a colonoscopy at the age of 50, which was normal. He was recommend to repeat the colonoscopy in 10 years, but he "can't find time" to schedule. Vaccinations are up to date, including tetanus, shingles, pneumococcal, hepatitis A and B, and annual influenza shots.

In the family, there is no known history of cardiac arrest, stroke, or blood clots. He is of Sicilian descent and his parents still live in Sicily; mother is 89 with HTN; father is 93 with DM, HTN, and emphysema. His brother is deceased (age 45, HTN, ruptured thoracic aortic aneurysm); sister is 60 with HTN and breast cancer. The patient's wife of 32 years is a registered dietician and they have no children. He works as a real estate agent for the past 35 years. He follows a strict exercise regimen, bicycling 20 miles a day, 7 days per week, for the last 15 years. A fear of sudden death, as in his brother, drives this passion. He drinks one glass of red wine with dinner 3 nights per week and denies ever using tobacco or recreational drugs.

ALLERGIES

No known drug allergies; no known food allergies.

MEDICATIONS

- Lisinopril 20 mg PO QD.
- Atorvastatin 40 mg PO QD.
- Cyclobenzaprine 10mg PO PRN.

PHYSICAL EXAMINATION

- *Vitals:* T 36.8°C (98.2°F), P 77, R 14, BP 110/78 mmg, SaO_2 97% RA, T 88.5 kg (195 lb), Ht 187.96 cm (74 in.), BMI 25.0.
- *General:* Well-developed, fit and healthy-appearing male, A&O×4, all vital signs stable. In no acute distress while seated upright and motionless; becomes acutely distressed with chest pain when supine.
- *Psychiatric:* Restricted affect, moderate psychomotor slowing, speech slow but coherent.
- *Skin:* Warm and dry with small bright red petechiae over medial-distal LLE along area of 1+ pitting edema that is mildly tender.
- *Chest:* No thoracic deformities or lesions, no increase in anteroposterior diameter. Chest wall markedly tender at right. proximal anterior axillary line.
- *Lungs:* Exam limited due to severe pain with deep breath; however, lungs are CTA with no adventitious sounds noted.
- *Heart:* RRR with no murmurs, gallops, or rubs. No displacement of PMI. No JVD noted.
- *Abdomen:* NABS in 4 quadrants with no bruits noted. Soft, nontender, nondistended; no masses, hepatosplenomegaly, or hernia present.
- *Musculoskeletal/extremities:* Distal LLE with 1+ tender pitting edema, and petechiae as noted above. Left ankle moderately edematous with passive FROM and no joint line tenderness. No clubbing or cyanosis.
- *Neurologic:* Gate slow and deliberate but steady; no tremors noted, 5/5 strength in BLE with sensation intact to light touch bilaterally.

CLINICAL DISCUSSION QUESTIONS

1. What is the differential diagnosis?

____

____

____

____

2. What is the most likely diagnosis? Why?

____

____

____

____

3. Demonstrate your understanding about pathophysiology of the most likely diagnosis.

4. Should tests/imaging studies be ordered? Which ones? Why? Think about tests/imaging beyond the primary care setting as well.

5. What are the next appropriate steps in management?

6. What are the risk predictors and symptom duration of the diagnosis? Provide references for your response.

7. What are the pertinent ICD-10 and CPT (E/M) codes for this visit? Provide a short rationale.

8. What is the appropriate patient education topic for this case?

9. If not managed appropriately, what is/are the medical/legal concern(s) that may arise?

10. Think about interprofessional collaboration for this case. Provide a list of specialties or other disciplines and indicate what contribution these professionals might make to managing the patient.

BEDSIDE MANNER QUESTION

11. What would your communication style/approach be with this patient?

Answers available at courseconnect.springerpub.com.

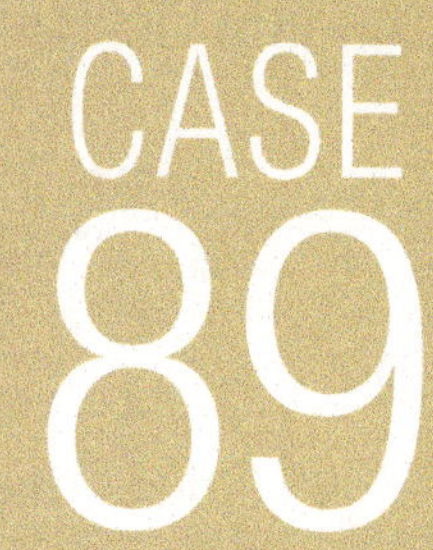

CASE 89

WELL VISIT, GERIATRIC MALE

Chief Complaint

"Adult well visit."

History of Present Illness

A 66-year-old man presents to his PCP for his annual adult well visit and a 6-month history of fatigue that he attributes to waking up 2 to 3 times a night to urinate. He is not too concerned because some of his friends experience similar symptoms. There have been no dietary, social, or environmental changes in his life during the past year. He is not taking any prescription or OTC medications. He states he generally feels well, exercises 3 times a week for 30 minutes a day, and eats healthy organic foods as much as possible. He has no chronic illnesses or relevant medical history.

Review of Systems

The patient's ROS is positive for mild fatigue, sleep disturbance, nocturia, decreased urinary stream, some urinary hesitancy, and occasional dribbling. His ROS is negative for fever, unexplained weight loss, SOB, polyuria, polydipsia, dysuria, hematuria, urethral discharge, urinary urgency, urinary frequency, and incontinence.

Relevant History

The patient's history is negative for major illnesses and trauma. As part of a comprehensive annual visit, a review of his last routine lab tests, colonoscopy, vision, and hearing tests are negative. His immunizations are up to date including tetanus, diphtheria, acellular pertussis, pneumococcal 13-valent conjugate (1 year ago), recombinant zoster, and influenza vaccines.

His social history includes drinking 1 to 2 beers per week since age 20 and an average of three cups of coffee per day. The patient has been a bodybuilder since his 30s, working out with weights three times a week. He and his husband walk 2 miles together on most mornings. HIV risk factors were assessed: The patient has one sex partner (husband) and engages in both insertive and receptive anal sex 2 to 3 times a week. His partner has no other sexual partners. A screen for STIs prior to their marriage 10 years ago was negative for gonorrhea, chlamydia, syphilis, hepatitis B, hepatitis C, and HIV. His family history is significant in that his father died of prostate cancer at 68 years of age. He has no uncles or brothers.

Allergies

No known drug allergies; no known food allergies.

Medications

None.

Physical Examination

- *Vitals:* T 37.0°C (98.6°F), P 76, R 14, BP 122/80 mmHg, HT 183 cm (72 in.), WT 82 kg (180.8 lb), BMI 24.5.
- *General:* Well-developed, well-nourished male in no acute distress.
- *Psychiatric:* Appears slightly anxious and somewhat fatigued.

- *Skin, Hair, and Nails:* No rashes or lesions. Hair and nails with no abnormal findings.
- *Eyes:* Vision 20/20 with corrective lenses on Snellen test.
- *ENT/Mouth:* Hearing grossly intact.
- *Neck:* Thyroid not enlarged, no palpable nodules.
- *Chest:* Chest expansion is symmetrical.
- *Heart:* RRR without murmur or gallop.
- *Lungs:* CTA bilaterally.
- *Abdomen:* Active BS; abdomen soft, nontender; no masses.
- *Genital/Rectal:* Uncircumcised male, no discharge or lesions, no scrotal or testicular masses. Soft, nontender, symmetrical, boggy, 2+ enlarged prostate, loss of median sulcus; no palpable prostate nodules.
- *Musculoskeletal:* No tenderness; FROM on BUE and BLE.
- *Neurologic:* A&O, CN II to XII intact.

Clinical Discussion Questions

1. What is the differential diagnosis?

2. What is the most likely diagnosis? Why?

3. Demonstrate your understanding about the pathophysiology of the most likely diagnosis.

4. Should tests/imaging studies be ordered? Which ones? Why? Think about tests/imaging beyond the primary care setting as well.

5. What are the next appropriate steps in management?

6. Discuss severity of symptoms, initial preferred treatment, how treatment can affect sexual function, and activities that can affect relevant blood tests for this diagnosis. Provide references to support your statements.

7. What are the pertinent ICD-10 and CPT (E/M) codes for this visit? Provide a short rationale.

8. What is the appropriate patient education topic for this case?

9. If not managed appropriately, what is/are the medical/legal concern(s) that may arise?

10. Think about interprofessional collaboration for this case. Provide a list of specialties or other disciplines and indicate what contribution these professionals might make to managing the patient.

BEDSIDE MANNER QUESTIONS

11. What would your communication style/approach be with this patient?

12. If a patient is distressed by the diagnosis, what might offer support?

Answers available at courseconnect.springerpub.com.

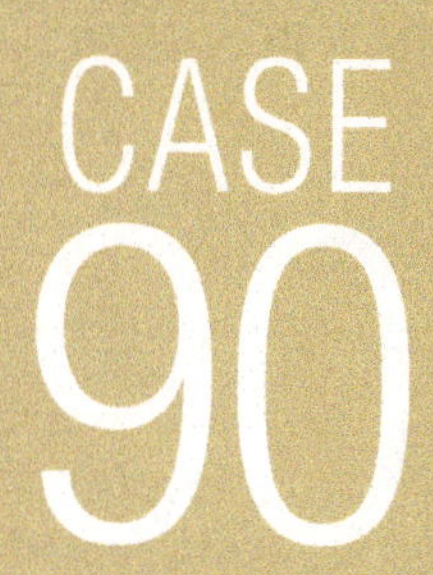

SHORTNESS OF BREATH, GERIATRIC MALE

Chief Complaint

"Shortness of breath."

History of Present Illness

A 74-year-old man presents for SOB, cough, wheezing, and fatigue for 1 week. His SOB and cough have worsened in the past 3 days, prompting him to seek care at the clinic. He denies fever, sweating, or chills. The patient states that he has been getting "winded" when he walks to his mailbox (approximately 60 ft./1.8m). On further questioning, the patient admits to smoking one pack of cigarettes a day for the past 50 years and has no desire to quit. He states, "I will die soon anyway, why quit now?" On further review of his patient chart, it is noted that he has presented with the same chief complaint in the past and was diagnosed with acute bronchitis and treated with albuterol and antibiotics. He has not been to the office in over 3 years.

Review of Systems

The patient's ROS is positive for productive cough, wheezing, SOB, fatigue, dyspnea on exertion, crackles, and clubbing of fingernails. His ROS is negative for fever, chills, adenopathy, cyanosis, pallor, palpitations, or barrel chest.

Relevant History

The patient has medically uncontrolled HTN and hyperlipidemia. He has been using albuterol and beclomethasone dipropionate inhaler occasionally for his SOB. He is not sure why he takes them. He denies having a history of asthma. He is a smoker. He has not received his flu vaccine for the last few years. He is not sure if he has ever had a pneumonia vaccine. He drinks about six 12-ounce beers three times a week. He is retired but used to work as an auto mechanic. No surgical history is reported. He does not know his family history.

Allergies

No known drug allergies; no known food allergies.

Medications

- Lisinopril 20 mg, QD
- Atorvastatin 20 mg, QD
- Albuterol 90 mcg inhaler, two puffs via inhalation Q4h PRN for chest tightness or cough.
- Beclomethasone dipropionate 80 mg inhaler, two puffs via inhalation Q12h.
- Ibuprofen 600 mg OTC, PRN for general aches.
- Guaifenesin cough syrup OTC, 15 mL Q6h PRN for cough.

Physical Examination

- *Vitals:* T 36.6°C (97.9°F), P 85, R 20, BP 152/88, SpO_2 93%, HT 180.3 cm (71 in.), WT 84.8 kg (187 lb), BMI 26.1.
- *General:* Appears to be in mild respiratory distress due to accessory muscle usage for breathing, not tripoding. Noted a thin body habitus.
- *Psychiatric:* Normal affect and judgment on exam.

- *Skin, Hair, and Nails:* Mild clubbing of nails noted. No pallor or cyanosis present.
- *ENT/Mouth:* Pink and moist oropharyngeal mucosa without exudates or lesions.
- *Neck:* Supple, no adenopathy noted.
- *Lungs:* Diffuse wheezing and crackles noted in both upper and lower lung fields. Labored breathing with accessory muscle usage noted; symmetrical expansion of lungs noted. Increased resonance to percussion noted. Decreased breath sounds throughout.
- *Heart:* RRR; no murmur or gallops.
- *Neurologic:* A&O×3, no focal deficit on exam noted.

Clinical Discussion Questions

1. What is the differential diagnosis?

2. What is the most likely diagnosis? Why?

3. Demonstrate your understanding about the pathophysiology of the most likely diagnosis.

4. Should tests/imaging studies be ordered? Which ones? Why? Think about tests/imaging beyond the primary care setting as well.

5. What are the next appropriate steps in management?

6. Review recent and credible research articles on this diagnosis. What is a common misdiagnosis and what are initial treatment options? Provide references for your response.

7. What are the pertinent ICD-10 and CPT (E/M) codes for this visit? Provide a short rationale.

8. What is the appropriate patient education topic for this case?

9. If not managed appropriately, what is/are the medical/legal concern(s) that may arise?

10. Think about interprofessional collaboration for this case. Provide a list of specialties or other disciplines and indicate what contribution these professionals might make to managing the patient.

BEDSIDE MANNER QUESTION

11. What would your communication style/approach be with this patient?

____

____

____

____

Answers available at courseconnect.springerpub.com.

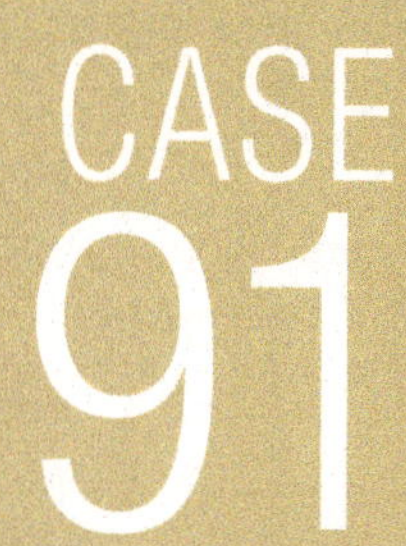

CASE 91

LIGHTHEADEDNESS, GERIATRIC FEMALE

Chief Complaint

"Lightheadedness."

History of Present Illness

A 68-year-old-woman with a medical history of essential HTN presents to her PCP with generalized weakness and lightheadedness. She states she has been unwell overall for the past 3 days. She is weak to the point of having a hard time performing the usual tasks around the house. The patient states she has been lying down for most of the past 2 days. When she gets up and walks around, she is intermittently lightheaded. She is overall active and usually enjoys working in her garden, but the past few days she has been unable to do so due to the fatigue and lightheadedness. The patient is generally adherent with her medications, which include hydrochlorothiazide 25 mg PO QD and amlodipine 5 mg PO QD. She is accompanied by her daughter who has reported that in addition to the fatigue, her mother has had a lack of appetite and decreased oral intake over the past 2 days.

Review of Systems

A directed ROS is positive for fatigue, fevers, chills, left-sided flank pain, dysuria, and urinary frequency. Her ROS is negative for headaches, visual disturbances, nasal congestion, sore throat, palpitations, chest pain, abdomen pain, nausea/vomiting, focal weakness or numbness, confusion, weight gain or loss, polyphagia or polydipsia, anxiety, or depression.

Relevant History

The patient's history is significant for essential HTN diagnosed at age 52; her social history is negative for drug, tobacco, or alcohol use. She reports a family history of HTN and high cholesterol. The patient lives at home with her husband, they have been married for 33 years, and she describes her marriage and family life as happy and healthy. She has two children who are both grown and living on their own.

Allergies

No known allergies; no known food allergies.

Medications

- Hydrochlorothiazide 25 mg PO QD.
- Amlodipine 5 mg PO QD.

Physical Examination

- *Vitals:* T 38.8°C (102°F), P 106, R 18, BP 88/30, HT 165.10 cm (65 in.), WT 61.2 kg (135 lb), BMI 22.5.
- *General:* Patient is in no apparent distress, appears stated age.
- *Psychiatric:* Normal affect, no disorganized behavior.
- *Skin, Hair, and Nails:* No rashes, normal skin turgor, normal hair texture, nails without splinter hemorrhages or clubbing.

- *Head:* Normocephalic, atraumatic, no lesions.
- *Eyes:* PERRL, anicteric sclerae.
- *ENT/Mouth:* Mucous membranes dry, no oral cavity lesions, oropharynx without erythema.
- *Neck:* Normal neck circumference, no thyromegaly.
- *Chest:* No obvious pectus deformity, normal excursion.
- *Lungs:* Unlabored respirations, CTA bilaterally.
- *Heart:* RRR, no murmurs, S1 and S2 present with normal timing.
- *Abdomen:* No striae, soft, nontender, BS are present and normoactive.
- *Musculoskeletal:* Left-sided costovertebral angle tenderness.
- *Neurologic:* A&O×3, CN II to XII intact, motor strength is 5/5 at the UE and BLE, no gross sensory deficits.

Clinical Discussion Questions

1. What is the differential diagnosis?

2. What is the most likely diagnosis? Why?

3. Demonstrate your understanding about the pathophysiology of the most likely diagnosis.

4. Should tests/imaging studies be ordered? Which ones? Why? Think about tests/imaging beyond the primary care setting as well.

5. What are the next appropriate steps in management?

6. Review a reliable, recent reference and demonstrate diagnostic criteria and treatment approach associated with this diagnosis. Include the name of the reference.

7. What are the pertinent ICD-10 and CPT (E/M) codes for this visit? Provide a short rationale.

8. What is the appropriate patient education topic for this case?

9. If not managed appropriately, what is/are the medical/legal concern(s) that may arise?

10. Think about interprofessional collaboration for this case. Provide a list of specialties or other disciplines and indicate what contribution these professionals might make to managing the patient.

BEDSIDE MANNER QUESTION

11. What would your communication/style approach be with this patient?

____

____

____

____

Answers available at courseconnect.springerpub.com.

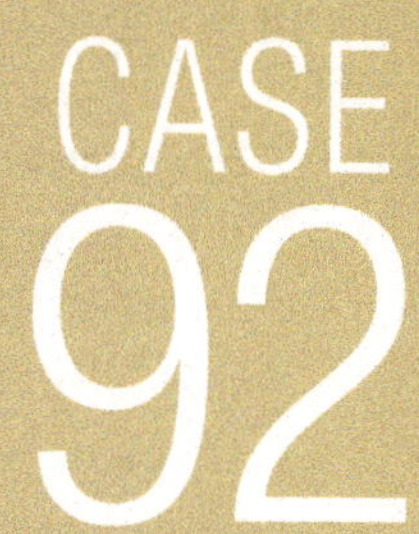

CASE 92

BUTTOCKS PAIN, GERIATRIC MALE

Chief Complaint

"Buttocks pain."

History of Present Illness

A 67-year-old man presents to establish care as a new patient. He has mental retardation, HTN, T2DM, and hyperlipidemia for which he has been off medication for 6 months. He complains of buttocks pain for a few days. He denies any falls.

He is living with his disabled sister and niece who have taken care of him for the last few years after they removed him from a residential facility due to cost. He was in a program that provided sheltered work experience and socialization. His niece is the patient's payee and manages his financial and medical needs; however, she has not taken him to a doctor for over 6 months and is not keeping him adherent to his medical regimen.

The patient's last Hgb A1C was 8.6% over 6 months ago, and he does not have a glucometer for BG monitoring. The dates of his last eye exam or dental exam are unknown.

His sister has limited ability to help the patient meet his medical and physical needs due to her medical condition. The niece is not interested in home health services. She uses the patient's and her mother's disability checks to pay for bills and does not have money left for medications.

The patient states he washes dishes and watches TV during the day for his activities. He is able to bathe and toilet himself with prompting and assistance. He uses a walker for stability with ambulation. He is missing his glasses and dentures due to frequent moves over the last few years.

Review of Systems

The patient's ROS is positive for weight loss of 20 lb, missing teeth, poor visual acuity, right shoulder pain with movement, right foot drop, and weakness. His ROS is negative for fever, chills, fatigue, vomiting, diarrhea, polyuria, polydipsia, and polyphagia. All other ROS are negative.

Relevant History

The patient's history is significant for intellectual disability, T2DM, HTN, hyperlipidemia, right foot drop, and nearsightedness. He had a full dental extraction in 2013. He lives with his sister, niece, and his niece's three children. He does not drink alcohol or use tobacco products or illicit drugs.

Allergies

No known drug allergies; no known food allergies.

Medications

- Enalapril 20 mg PO BID.
- Glipizide 5 mg PO BID.
- Metformin 1000 mg PO BID.
- Metoprolol tartrate 50 mg PO BID.
- Pravastatin 40 mg PO QD.

PHYSICAL EXAMINATION

- *Vitals:* T 37°C (98.6°F), P 88, R 16, BP 180/100, HT 185.4 cm (73 in.), WT 126.6 kg (279 lb), BMI 36.81.
- *General:* Well-developed, malnourished appearing 67-year-old man in acute distress. Poor hygiene with dirty clothes and foul body odor. Able to answer questions.
- *Psychiatric:* Normal mood.
- *Skin, Hair, and Nails:* Dry appearing, macerated, erythematous skin on buttocks and gluteal fold with dry fecal material. Partial thickness, loss of dermis with shallow ulceration on left buttocks. Dirty, long fingernails. Toenails are thickened and yellow with extensive growth needing trimming to normal length.
- *ENT/Mouth:* Dry oral mucosa, teeth are absent, no dentures.
- *Lungs:* CTA bilaterally.
- *Heart:* RRR, without murmur, gallop, or rub.
- *Abdomen:* Soft, nondistended. NABS are heard in all four quadrants.
- *Musculoskeletal:* No joint swelling or pain. Wide gait with dragging of right foot.
- *Neurologic:* Coordination abnormal with drop foot pattern of right foot. Sensory exam of the foot is abnormal with monofilaments in all locations. Weak pulses, no lesions, or ulcers. Mini-cog was normal.

CLINICAL DISCUSSION QUESTIONS

1. What is the differential diagnosis?

____

____

____

____

2. What is the most likely diagnosis? Why?

____

____

____

____

3. Demonstrate your understanding about the pathophysiology of the most likely diagnosis.

____

____

____

____

4. Should tests/imaging studies be ordered? Which ones? Why? Think about tests/imaging beyond the primary care setting as well.

5. What are the next appropriate steps in management?

6. What are the risk factors, clinical presentation, and PCP responsibility associated with the diagnosis? Provide references for your response.

7. What are the pertinent ICD-10 and CPT (E/M) codes for this visit? Provide a short rationale.

8. What is the appropriate patient/caregiver education topic for this case?

9. If not managed appropriately, what is/are the medical/legal concern(s) that may arise?

10. Think about interprofessional collaboration for this case. Provide a list of specialties or other disciplines and indicate what contribution these professionals might make to managing the patient.

BEDSIDE MANNER QUESTION

11. What would your communication style/approach be with this patient and family?

Answers available at courseconnect.springerpub.com.

URINE LEAKAGE, GERIATRIC FEMALE

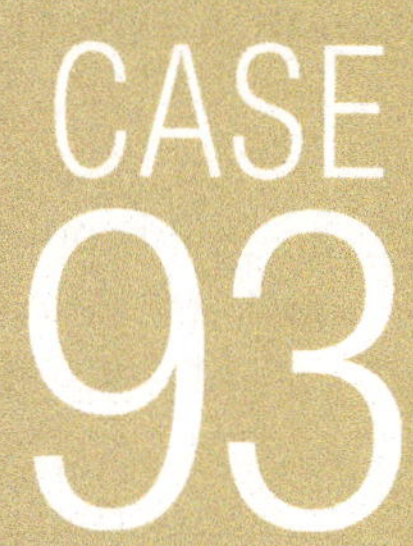

Chief Complaint

"Urine leakage."

History of Present Illness

A 66-year-old White woman presents with complaints of "leaking urine" and urgency of urination for 6 to 12 months. These symptoms have persisted to the point that she has identified every public bathroom between her home and work and developed clear preferences for bathrooms in certain gas stations and fast food establishments. When she enters a new restaurant, she instinctively looks for the bathroom before being seated. Her concern is that when she is struck with the urge to urinate, she begins to leak, and she may not have more than a minute to get to the bathroom before she has an "accident." She experiences urinary frequency 8 to 10 times daily, often with episodes of leaking and occasionally with nocturia. She rates the symptoms as 7 of 10 on a bother scale.

Pelvic floor–strengthening exercises (Kegel exercises) and OTC herbal remedies have not helped. She experiences limited benefit from fluid restriction and is careful to urinate at home before driving. She wears incontinence pads to avoid the embarrassment of leaking and soiling her clothes in public.

Review of Systems

The ROS is positive for fatigue, nausea, abdominal pain, and hematuria. The patient reported headache and dizziness. The ROS is negative for fever, chills, glaucoma, vomiting, diarrhea, constipation, SOB, or chest pain.

Relevant History

Medical history is significant for Cesarean section (age 34) and a total hysterectomy (age 51) for menorrhagia. Her social history includes drinking one glass of wine per week since age 20, and she does not use recreational drugs. She admits to smoking a half pack of cigarettes per day for the last 10 years. Her two children are grown and have families of their own. She has suffered from intermittent depression since her husband died 8 years ago. Her family history is unremarkable.

Allergies

No known drug allergies; no known food allergies.

Medications

- Acetaminophen 500 mg PRN for arthralgia.
- Magnesium 250 mg nightly for sleep.
- Calcium 1,200 mg QD.
- Vitamin D 600 IU QD.
- Multivitamin QD.

Physical Examination

- *Vitals:* T 36.9°C (98.4°F), P 76, R 14, BP 122/78, HT 168 cm (66 in.), WT 86 kg (189.5 lb), BMI 30.5.
- *General:* Well-developed, well-nourished, obese woman in no acute distress.

- *Psychiatric:* Judgment and insight intact; rate of thoughts normal and logical; pleasant, calm, and cooperative; patient appears to be happy and content without overt anxiety or depression.
- *Abdomen:* Active BS; abdomen soft, nontender; no masses, no hernias, no suprapubic distension.
- *Genital/Rectal:* No bladder tenderness on palpation and no distention noted. Atrophic external genitalia without prolapse, pelvic masses, or gross lesions. Vagina mucosa exhibits thinning and pallor with loss of rugae. No urinary leakage on cough test with a full bladder. On the rectal exam, perineal sensation intact; sphincter tone intact; able to contract the anal sphincter.
- *Neurologic:* A&O×3; CN grossly intact; communication ability within normal limits; attention and concentration normal; sensation to light touch is intact; gait is within normal limits for age.

CLINICAL DISCUSSION QUESTIONS

1. What is the differential diagnosis?

2. What is the most likely diagnosis? Why?

3. Demonstrate your understanding about the pathophysiology of the most likely diagnosis.

4. Should tests/imaging studies be ordered? Which ones? Why? Think about tests/imaging beyond the primary care setting as well.

5. What are the next appropriate steps in management?

6. Review recent and credible research article(s) on this diagnosis. What are the helpful tools for making the diagnosis and treatment options? List your reference(s).

7. What are the pertinent ICD-10 and CPT (E/M) codes for this visit? Provide a short rationale.

8. What is the appropriate patient education topic for this case?

9. If not managed appropriately, what is/are the medical/legal concern(s) that may arise?

10. Think about interprofessional collaboration for this case. Provide a list of specialties or other disciplines and indicate what contribution these professionals might make to managing the patient.

BEDSIDE MANNER QUESTION

11. What would your communication style/approach be with this patient?

____

____

____

____

Answers available at courseconnect.springerpub.com.

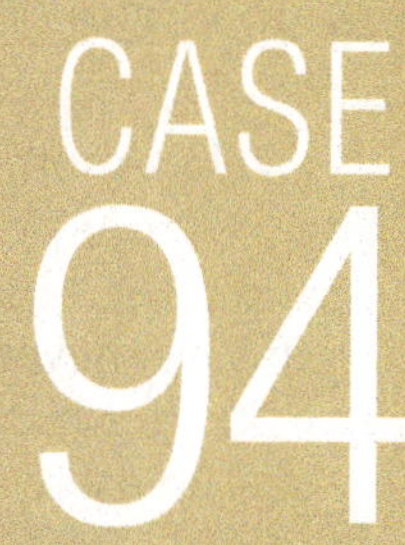

CONFUSION, GERIATRIC FEMALE

Chief Complaint

"Confusion."

History of Present Illness

An 80-year-old woman with mild Parkinson disease, severe GAD, GERD, and chronic urinary retention with recurrent UTIs is brought in to her PCP's office by her daughter because of mild confusion over the past 2 days. The daughter has observed her compulsively taking her temperature and wandering around the house, repeatedly stating, "Am I septic?" The patient, who is typically sharp and lucid, called her PCP 2 weeks ago complaining of urinary urgency and incontinence but refused an office visit or urine test because she was "too busy" with other appointments. Considering her history and upon review of her most recent urine culture and sensitivity testing performed 2 months prior, a prescription for nitrofurantoin was called in to her pharmacy, she was given ED precautions, and she was advised to schedule a follow-up appointment in 1 week.

Today, the patient states she did not come in because her urinary symptoms improved, but she admits she feels worse overall, endorsing nausea, anorexia, weight loss, diffuse body aches, chills, and night sweats, which she attributes to her new medication for PD, which was started 6 months ago. She denies dysuria, hematuria, fever, or flank pain but notes she "never has" dysuria with her UTIs. "I just shiver when I get the enterococcus; that's how I know it's not the *E. coli*." She asks repeatedly "Do I have sepsis?" because home temperature "always runs 96.8," which is "too low" according to her internet research. She has not returned to her urologist in over a year. "He just wants to give me another pill; I won't take it."

The patient's daughter, who works two jobs and is not home much, states that the patient is not compliant with prescribed medications, even with a pill box. The patient carefully reads all pharmacy package inserts, gets scared by the lists of side effects, and then searches the internet to see how "dangerous" the medication is before deciding whether she will take it. The patient admits she cuts most pills in half or takes less than the prescribed dose because she is "allergic to everything." The patient states she only took the nitrofurantoin pill once a day instead of BID and for only 4 of the 7 days prescribed. "I hate that pill. I get so nauseated." She does not trust prescription medications in general. "I read the internet, I know about pharma, I want natural antibiotics, D-mannose, cranberry."

Review of Systems

The patient's ROS is positive for chills, weight loss, fatigue, constipation, rectal wipe-bleeding and rectal discomfort "when hemorrhoids swell," insomnia, depression, and anxiety. It is positive for vaginal itching and pain, chronic, without discharge or bleeding. It is positive for skin itching "all over" but no rash. Her ROS is negative for fever. She has no cough, SOB, or dyspnea on exertion. It is negative for chest pain, palpitations, dizziness, or edema; abdominal pain, vomiting, or melena; weakness, paresthesia, or dysarthria; or forgetfulness or getting lost.

Relevant History

In addition to PD, severe GAD, GERD, and chronic urinary retention/recurrent UTIs, the patient has essential HTN, hyperlipidemia, impaired fasting glucose, gout, hypothyroidism, hearing loss (refuses hearing aids), and allergic rhinitis.

The patient underwent open cholecystectomy in 1967, thyroidectomy in 1978, and TAH/BSO in 1985, all for benign conditions. She absolutely refuses mammograms, colon cancer screening, and vaccinations, due to fear of side effects.

Her mother died at 71 from heart disease; her father died at 90 from "old age." Her brother died at 78 from prostate cancer, and one daughter, age 54, has bipolar disorder. The patient is a widow and retired high school teacher with a master's degree; she drinks one glass of wine once per week and has never smoked or used recreational drugs. She moved in with her daughter 10 years ago, when her husband died, and does not drive due to anxiety. She eats "whatever sounds good" and gets no exercise other than going to her appointments and has no outside interest or hobbies.

ALLERGIES

No known drug allergies; no known food allergies.

MEDICATIONS

- Prescribed medications include the following:
  - Levothyroxine 100 mcg QD
  - Allopurinol 100 mg QD
  - Metoprolol succinate ER 25 mg QD
  - Carbidopa-levodopa 25 mg/100 mg TID
  - Vitamin D 2000 IU QD
  - Polyethylene glycol 3350 17 g in 8 oz fluid QD
  - Loratadine 10 mg QD
  - Diazepam 2 mg BID PRN for anxiety/insomnia
- She has been using an expired prescription for triamcinolone acetonide 0.1% cream on her vulva BID for itching for the last 6 months.
- She continues to take conjugated estrogens 0.3 mg PO QD prescribed by her urologist.
- She has stopped all GERD medications because they give her a headache.

PHYSICAL EXAMINATION

- *Vitals:* T 36.7°C (98.1°F), P 74, R 14, BP 132/60, SpO_2 98%, HT 160 cm (63 in.), WT 89.8 kg. (198 lb), BMI 35.1 (weight down 3 lb in 5 months).
- *General:* Well-developed, well-appearing, overnourished older female, A&O×3. All vital signs stable. In no acute distress; ate entire bag of chips and drank one can of a nutrition supplement during interview.
- *Psychiatric:* Labile affect, pressured and tangential speech with logorrhea (no change from patient's baseline); fair insight.
- *Skin, Hair, and Nails:* Warm and dry, no rashes noted on full skin exam. Moist, sticky intertriginous areas present in inframammary, intergluteal, and inguinal regions. No abnormal findings with hair or nails.
- *Lungs:* CTA bilaterally with no adventitious sounds noted.
- *Heart:* RRR with no murmurs, gallops, or rubs.
- *Abdomen:* NABS in four quadrants with no bruits noted. Soft, nontender, nondistended; no masses, hepatosplenomegaly, or hernia present. Surgical scars at RUQ and midline lower are well healed. No costovertebral angle tenderness elicited.
- *Genital/Rectal:* External genitalia, Bartholin glands, urethra, and Skene glands fully obscured by talcum powder; vaginal mucosa pink but extremely dry and thin with no abnormal discharge noted. Swab of vaginal vault obtained for wet mount. Tender anal canal with multiple moderate-sized nonthrombosed external and internal hemorrhoids and no fissures noted; tan soft stool in vault; heme negative.
- *Musculoskeletal:* Good muscle tone; no clubbing or cyanosis; radial pulses 2+ bilaterally.
- *Neurologic:* Slow but steady gait without shuffling; no tremors or cogwheeling noted; 5/5 strength BLEs with sensation intact to light touch bilaterally. Gross hearing decreased bilaterally. MMSE score 27/30.

CLINICAL DISCUSSION QUESTIONS

1. What is the differential diagnosis?

2. What is the most likely diagnosis? Why?

3. Demonstrate your understanding about the pathophysiology of the most likely diagnosis.

4. Should tests/imaging studies be ordered? Which ones? Why? Think about tests/imaging beyond the primary care setting as well.

5. What are the next appropriate steps in management?

6. What is the clinical presentation of the older adult, and what is the initial treatment associated with the diagnosis? Provide references for your response.

7. What are the pertinent ICD-10 and CPT (E/M) codes for this visit? Provide a short rationale.

8. What is the appropriate patient education topic for this case?

9. If not managed appropriately, what is/are the medical/legal concern(s) that may arise?

10. Think about interprofessional collaboration for this case. Provide a list of specialties or other disciplines and indicate what contribution these professionals might make to managing the patient.

BEDSIDE MANNER QUESTION

11. What would your communication style/approach be with this patient?

Answers available at courseconnect.springerpub.com.

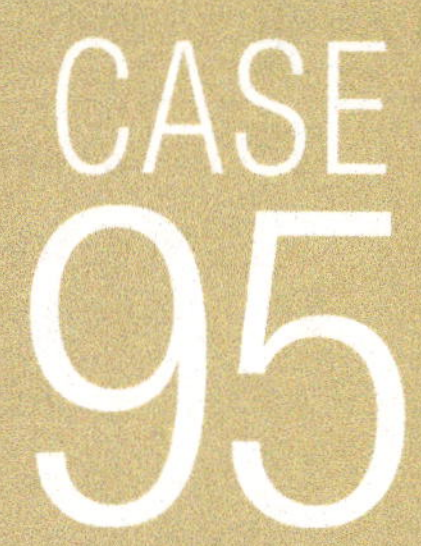

CASE 95

LEG PAIN, GERIATRIC MALE

Chief Complaint

"Leg pain."

History of Present Illness

A 74-year-old man, well established in this primary care clinic, presents complaining of leg pain that has been bothering him for the past few months. He states that the 4/10, crampy calf pain in both legs occurs about 15 minutes into his BID walks with his dog. The pain only goes away when he stops walking and sits for about 5 minutes. Once he starts walking again, the pain returns just a few minutes later. He also states that his legs feel weak. He reports pain relief upon elevating his legs while relaxing in his recliner but reports he sometimes cannot sleep at night as his legs start cramping when he lies down. He feels he cannot hold them still because the pain at times becomes an intense 6/10 to 7/10 until he falls asleep. He denies taking any medications for this pain but states standing in one place for an extended period, such as when fishing, also makes the pain return.

Review of Systems

The patient's ROS is positive for leg cramps and weakness, varicose veins, and arthritis in hands and feet. His ROS is negative for fainting, blackouts, seizures, weakness, paralysis, tingling, tremors, or erectile dysfunction. He denies chest pain, palpitations, dyspnea at rest or upon exertion, orthopnea, paroxysmal nocturnal dyspnea, edema, and any recent trauma to his lower extremities.

Relevant History

The patient has hypercholesterolemia, HTN, and BL cataracts with lens implants. The patient is a retired engineer, happily married to his wife of 54 years. He is a former tobacco abuser, 2 packs per day for 30 years; he quit at age 48. He enjoys two martinis with dinner each evening and denies recreational or illicit drug use ever. His family history is significant for lung cancer, acute MI, hyperlipidemia, and HTN.

Allergies

No known drug allergies; no known food allergies.

Medications

- Atorvastatin 40 mg PO QHS.
- Amlodipine 5 mg PO QD.

Physical Examination

- *Vitals:* T 36.9°C (98.4°F), P 78, R 14, BP 146/88, HT 178 cm (70 in.), WT 82.6 kg (182 lb), BMI 26.1.
- *General:* Pleasant male of stated age sitting comfortably on the examination table, in no acute distress. Makes good eye contact, converses with ease, makes jokes. A&O.
- *Skin, Hair, and Nails:* Tight, thin, shiny, atrophied skin, slightly dusky red/ruborous color, overlying dorsum of mid-feet to include all toes, extending proximally and circumferentially to BL ankles and knees. Bald, slightly cool to the touch bilaterally and symmetrically. No lesions or masses. Thin, short brittle nails BL feet.

- *Head:* Atraumatic, normocephalic.
- *Neck:* Trachea midline, no masses or lymphadenopathy.
- *Lungs:* CTA bilaterally without wheezes or rales.
- *Heart:* RRR; no murmurs, rubs, or gallops.
- *Peripheral Vascular:* Carotid pulses 2+ bilaterally; no thrills or bruits. Distal upper extremity pulses 2+ and symmetric bilaterally, capillary refill <2 seconds. Distal lower extremity pulses: femoral and popliteal pulses 1+ symmetric bilaterally, posterior tibial pulses 1+ symmetric bilaterally. Dorsalis pedis pulses weak bilaterally with sluggish capillary refill. Spider vein varicosities throughout BLEs. With patient lying supine, great toes blanch while lower extremities are extended and held superiorly to approximately 60°. When lower extremities are returned to the supine position, the great toes return to their original dusky red color/ rubor within 6 seconds.
- *Musculoskeletal:* FROM BUEs. LROM BL feet and ankles, lower extremity muscle atrophy bilaterally, most notably BL calves distal to feet.
- *Neurologic:* CN II to XII grossly intact. Negative Romberg, antalgic gait with heel-to-toe walking, walking on heels, and walking on toes.

CLINICAL DISCUSSION QUESTIONS

1. What is the differential diagnosis?

2. What is the most likely diagnosis? Why?

3. Demonstrate your understanding about the pathophysiology of the most likely diagnosis.

4. Should tests/imaging studies be ordered? Which ones? Why? Think about tests/imaging beyond the primary care setting as well.

5. What are the next appropriate steps in management?

6. What is the prevalence of the diagnosis? What is the initial diagnostic procedure for this condition? What are the treatments? Provide references for your responses.

7. What are the pertinent ICD-10 and CPT (E/M) codes for this visit? Provide a short rationale.

8. What is the appropriate patient education topic for this case?

9. If not managed appropriately, what is/are the medical/legal concern(s) that may arise?

10. Think about interprofessional collaboration for this case. Provide a list of specialties or other disciplines and indicate what contribution these professionals might make to managing the patient.

BEDSIDE MANNER QUESTION

11. What would your communication style/approach be with this patient?

____

____

____

____

Answers available at courseconnect.springerpub.com.

SHORTNESS OF BREATH WITH EXERTION, GERIATRIC MALE

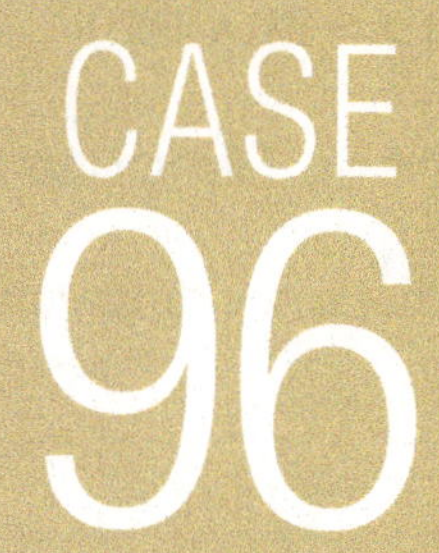

Chief Complaint

"SOB with exertion."

History of Present Illness

A 67-year-old male presents to clinic with a 2-month history of progressive SOB with exertion, nonproductive cough, and early satiety. He states that he initially noticed these symptoms almost a year ago when he would get full quickly and be unable to finish his entire meal. He would have subsequent heartburn symptoms and some acid reflux and occasionally regurgitate undigested food. However, over the past few months, he has had progressive SOB with activity. He does admit waking occasionally at night short of breath.

He denies any significant weight loss, infectious symptoms, any recent travel, fatigue, night sweats, wheezing, or hemoptysis. He is a lifetime nonsmoker and denies any occupational exposures or history of asthma. Of note, he does live in the California Central Valley. Cancer screening and all other recommendations are up to date.

Review of Systems

The patient's ROS is positive for dyspnea on exertion, GERD symptoms, nausea, occasional emesis, and night-time waking. ROS is negative for any fevers, sweats, chills, headaches, dizziness, lightheadedness, diarrhea, constipation, or dysuria. The patient also denies any chest pain, unintentional weight loss, or night sweats.

Relevant History

The patent's medical history is significant for HTN. He is a retired manager and lives at home with his wife and has 6 grandchildren. His family history is unknown.

Allergies

No known drug allergies; no known food allergies.

Medications

Losartan 50 mg PO QD.

Physical Examination

- *Vitals:* T 37°C (98.6°F), P 96, R 18, BP 136/84 mmHg, HT 172.7 cm (68 in.), WT 72.6 kg (160 lb), BMI 24.3.
- *General:* Nontoxic appearing, no acute distress.
- *Lungs:* Normal inspiratory effort. BS heard in left lower lung field.
- *Heart:* RRR, no murmurs, rubs or gallops.
- *Abdomen:* Nondistended, nontender to palpation. Positive BS in all 4 quadrants.
- *Musculoskeletal:* FROM in all extremities.

CLINICAL DISCUSSION QUESTIONS

1. What is the differential diagnosis?

2. What is the most likely diagnosis? Why?

3. Demonstrate your understanding about pathophysiology of the most likely diagnosis.

4. Should tests/imaging studies be ordered? Which ones? Why? Think about tests/imaging beyond the primary care setting as well.

5. What are the next appropriate steps in management?

6. What are the causes, comorbidities, incidence, and treatment options for this diagnosis? Provide references for your response.

7. What are the pertinent ICD-10 and CPT (E/M) codes for this visit? Provide a short rationale.

8. What is the appropriate patient education topic for this case?

9. If not managed appropriately, what is/are the medical/legal concern(s) that may arise?

10. Think about interprofessional collaboration for this case. Provide a list of specialties or other disciplines and indicate what contribution these professionals might make to managing the patient.

BEDSIDE MANNER QUESTION

11. What would your communication style/approach be with this patient?

____

____

____

____

Answers available at courseconnect.springerpub.com.

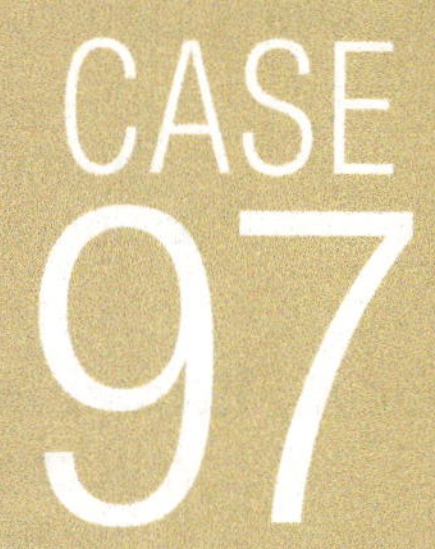

SCALP PAIN, GERIATRIC FEMALE

Chief Complaint

"It hurts to brush my hair."

History of Present Illness

A 74-year-old White woman presents to the primary care office with a complaint of scalp pain that has become worse over the past 5 days. She first noticed the pain around her temples and the top of her scalp, which she described as one of her typical headaches that occurs for a day or so—constant, not throbbing, and burning in nature anytime she brushes her hair. She states the pain has now radiated into the sides of her face, into the joints of her jaw and down into her shoulders, which has never happened before. She also reports feeling tired over these past few days, with not much stamina to do simple house chores, and noticed right-sided visual floaters have been occurring with more frequency. Although she admits to having "years" of periodic headaches, she has never sought medical attention for them and denies ever having symptoms quite like this. She does not recall anything that could have brought this on other than a prolonged dental appointment a day or so before her symptoms started.

Review of Systems

The patient's ROS is positive for fatigue; malaise; headaches; visual spots, specks, and floaters; and scalp, temple, facial, jaw, and shoulder pain/stiffness. Her ROS is negative for unintentional weight loss, insomnia, fever, chills, diaphoresis, double or loss of vision, congestion, trouble swallowing, chest pain, heart palpitations, dyspnea, lightheadedness, weakness, paresthesia, change in memory, and syncope or near syncope.

Relevant History

The patient has a past medical history significant for HTN, hyperlipidemia, BL carotid stenosis, and osteopenia. A BL carotid US performed 8 months ago demonstrated 35% stenosis of the left common carotid artery and 45% stenosis of the right common carotid artery. She had a laparoscopic cholecystectomy at age 46 and BL bunionectomies at age 50. She has never used tobacco products, drinks a glass of white wine socially once or twice per week, and does not use recreational or illicit drugs. Her diet consists of chicken, fish, vegetables, and fruit, as she is trying to maintain a healthy diet with low-sodium choices. She lives with her husband of 53 years and their dog, whom she walks twice per day for exercise.

The patient's family history is significant for HTN and carotid artery disease and CAD in her mother and hyperlipidemia and HTN in her father. Her parents are both deceased due to injuries sustained in an MVA; mother was 81 and father was 83. She has one brother, alive at age 76 with HTN, hyperlipidemia, and CAD and has sustained one MI several years ago. She has two adult children, both daughters, ages 49 and 46, both alive with HTN and hyperlipidemia.

Allergies

No known drug allergies; no known food allergies.

Medications

- Hydrochlorothiazide 25 mg PO BID.
- Amlodipine 10 mg PO QD.
- Aspirin 81 mg PO QD.

- Atorvastatin 40 mg PO QHS.
- Calcium citrate/vitamin D3 600 mg/800 IU PO BID.

PHYSICAL EXAMINATION

- *Vitals:* T 37.7°C (99.8°F), P 84, R 12, BP 152/86, and BMI 20.4, visual acuity 20/25 OD, 20/30 OS, 20/30 OU without corrective lenses.
- *General:* Elderly woman who appears her stated age, squinting her eyes in obvious discomfort as she rubs both temples while sitting on the examination table.
- *Psychiatric:* A&O×3.
- *Skin, Hair, and Nails:* Full head of thinning, white hair that when moved, elicits scalp pain. (-) lesions or rashes.
- *Head:* Atraumatic, normocephalic. Severe tenderness throughout forehead, anterior scalp distal to occiput, and BL temporal and parietal regions. (+) visible, nodular, tender right superficial temporal artery swelling, (-) swelling of left superficial temporal artery.
- *Eyes:* Sclera injected, nonicteric, (+) PERRLA, (+) EOMI, (-) retinal hemorrhage, A-V nicking, venous pulsations, optic disk cupping, papilledema.
- *ENT/Mouth:* (+) Severe tenderness of frontal and maxillary sinuses, TM joints bilaterally, (-) clicks but (+) increased pain upon mandible opening, closing, protrusion, talking. (-) TMJ swelling. Teeth in good condition, gingiva without lesions or abscess; moist, patent oropharynx with uvula midline.
- *Neck:* Supple, slight adenopathy. (+) carotid artery bruits bilaterally. (-) JVD, goiter. Trachea midline.
- *Lungs:* CTA bilaterally, (-) wheezes, rhonchi.
- *Heart:* RRR, (+) S1/S2, (-) murmurs, rubs, gallops.
- *Abdomen:* Flat, (+) BS × 4, soft, nontender. (-) aorta, BL renal, iliac and femoral artery thrills or bruits.
- *Peripheral vascular:* 2+ symmetric pulses UE and LE bilaterally. Cap refill < 2 sec throughout.
- *Musculoskeletal:* C-spine ROM 45° flexion, extension, 35° bending, 60° L and R rotation; BL shoulders ROM to 45° extension, 120° forward flexion of 120°, internal rotation 90°, very limited external rotation at 40°. (-) AP chest tenderness. (-) upper extremity joint swelling.
- *Neurologic:* (+) Severe pain, CNV with sharp/dull discrimination, all 3 divisions bilaterally, CN VII, CN XI, CN XII motor intact but equally painful. Remainder CNs grossly intact.

CLINICAL DISCUSSION QUESTIONS

1. What is the differential diagnosis?

____

____

____

____

2. What is the most likely diagnosis? Why?

____

____

____

____

3. Demonstrate your understanding about the pathophysiology of the most likely diagnosis.

4. Should tests/imaging studies be ordered? Which ones? Why? Think about tests/imaging beyond the primary care setting as well.

5. What are the next appropriate steps in management?

6. What are the diagnostic approach and risk factors for this diagnosis? Provide references for your response.

7. What are the pertinent ICD-10 and CPT (E/M) codes for this visit? Provide a short rationale.

8. What is the appropriate patient education topic for this case?

9. If not managed appropriately, what is/are the medical/legal concern(s) that may arise?

10. Think about interprofessional collaboration for this case. Provide a list of specialties or other disciplines and indicate what contribution these professionals might make to managing the patient.

BEDSIDE MANNER QUESTIONS

11. How would you communicate your likely diagnosis to the patient?

12. If the patient shows distress at what you communicate, how would you provide reassurance?

13. If diagnostic evidence points to a more complicated case that could potentially result in a negative outcome, how would you communicate this possibility?

Answers available at courseconnect.springerpub.com.

SHAKING HANDS, GERIATRIC MALE

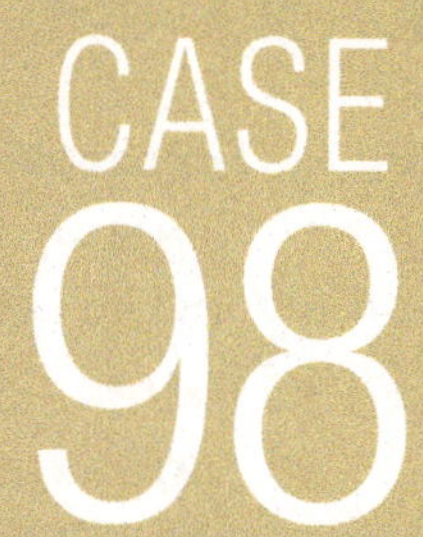

Chief Complaint

"Shaking hands."

History of Present Illness

A 67-year-old man presents to the primary care office for evaluation of "shaking hands." The patient first noticed it 4 years ago but it has progressively worsened since that time. He decided to be seen today because his family and friends have noticed the shaking as well. He states that the onset was gradual and has been slowly worsening over time. Initially, only the right hand was shaking, but now both hands are shaking. Stress and fatigue exacerbate the symptoms, as well as activities such as writing and handling objects. Alleviating factors include relaxing and not using his hands and when he takes the medication he is prescribed for his anxiety. His established psychiatrist has been managing his anxiety disorder. There is no additional limb involvement outside of the hands. The tremor is present throughout the day. He rates the severity at an 8 out of 10; he has become increasingly self-conscious of the shaking, and he states it has significantly impacted his daily activities including using utensils to eat his meals.

Review of Systems

The patient's ROS is positive for anxiety and difficulty sleeping for many years. ROS is negative for depression, changes in weight or appetite, or fatigue. Negative for trauma or recent falls, weakness, paresthesia, numbness, gait changes, or difficulty maintaining balance.

Relevant History

- The patient's medical history is significant for anxiety and insomnia diagnosed in his 30s.
- The patient's social history shows no current or previous smoking or tobacco use, no current or previous illicit drug use, and no current alcohol use. The patient's social history is significant for previous heavy alcohol use, from age 17 through 55. He has been abstinent from alcohol for 12 years and actively participates in Alcoholics Anonymous. He runs courses and support sessions for groups of people in recovery. He has been divorced for 15 years and currently lives alone.
- The patient's family history is significant for his father having a similar tremor which started in his late 70s; his father is now deceased (age 87, pneumonia). The patient denies any family history of neurologic disorders.

Allergies

No know drug allergies; no known food allergies.

Medications

- Alprazolam, 0.25 mg, 1 tablet PO PRN for anxiety and insomnia.
- Fluoxetine 20 mg, 1 tablet PO QD.

PHYSICAL EXAMINATION

- *Vitals:* T 37°C (98.6°F), P 82, R 14, BP 128/82 mmHg, HT 70 in. (177.8 cm), WT: 184 lb (83.46 kg), BMI 26.4.
- *General:* Well-appearing 67-year-old male in no acute distress.
- *Psychiatric:* Follows commands fully, cooperative with exam, provides full history without hesitation; clean, A&O×3, affect full and appropriate.
- *Skin, Hair, and Nails:* Skin intact without sloughing or dry patches.
- *ENT/Mouth:* EOMI in six cardinal positions of gaze, audible volume of speech, rhythmic voice shaking noted.
- *Musculoskeletal:* 5/5 strength in BL UEs and LEs; no atrophy of musculature; no reduced ROM.
- *Neurologic:*
  - DTRs 2+ equal and symmetrical in BL UEs and LEs. Negative glabellar reflex.
  - No increased or decreased tone through passive motion in BL UEs and LEs; negative for rigidity.
  - No tremor noted at rest; BL oscillating hand tremor noted in both hands when held up against gravity; tremor improves with weight and worsens at terminal goal-oriented activities (point-to-point assessment). No cogwheeling seen.
  - Rises from the chair easily without use of hands, negative retropulsion, symmetrical stride length without shuffling; spontaneous BL arm swing during ambulation.
  - Negative Romberg test.
  - RAMs intact.
  - Sensation intact to light and sharp touch on plantar surfaces of feet bilaterally.
  - Writing assessment: handwriting is normal size, but shaky (patient's rendition of spiral drawing test showed irregular lines that oscillated with the hand movement); intact BLE.
  - MMSE Score: 30/30.

CLINICAL DISCUSSION QUESTIONS

1. What is the differential diagnosis?

___

___

___

___

2. What is the most likely diagnosis? Why?

___

___

___

___

3. Demonstrate your understanding about the pathophysiology of the most likely diagnosis.

4. Should tests/imaging studies be ordered? Which ones? Why? Think about tests/imaging beyond the primary care setting as well.

5. What are the next appropriate steps in management?

6. Review credible research article(s) on this diagnosis. List your findings of the prevalence, preventive measures, and treatment options. Provide your reference(s).

7. What are the pertinent ICD-10 and CPT (E/M) codes for this visit? Provide a short rationale.

8. What is the appropriate patient education topic for this case?

9. If not managed appropriately, what is/are the medical/legal concern(s) that may arise?

10. Think about interprofessional collaboration for this case. Provide a list of specialties or other disciplines and indicate what contribution these professionals might make to managing the patient.

Bedside Manner Question

11. What would your communication style/approach be with this patient and his mother?

Answers available at courseconnect.springerpub.com.

FATIGUE, GERIATRIC FEMALE

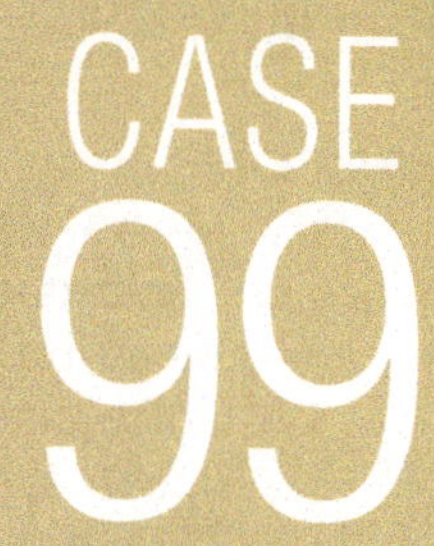

Chief Complaint

"I'm so tired."

History of Present Illness

A 74-year-old woman presents to her PCP complaining of increased fatigue, SOB, and a clear productive cough that has steadily worsened over the past 2 months. She reports slight lightheadedness and diaphoresis but denies fever or chills, stating her symptoms seem related to her seasonal allergies.

The patient reports an unintentional weight gain of 15 lb (6.8 kg) over the past 2 months, which she says she does not understand as she always feels full as well as constipated and she does not eat much. She has been trying to lose weight as she reports she cannot fasten her pants after dinner. She has been trying to participate in an exercise class with others her age, but she states she has no energy. She says it is exhausting just to park her car and walk into her exercise class from the parking lot. She attributes seasonal allergies to her hacking, productive cough, and fatigue, stating "it is a very, very hot summer, worse than usual." She also reports not sleeping well since her husband recently passed away. She was his sole caretaker for close to 9 years as he battled dementia and PD. She has been taking a prescribed sleep aid with more regularity but feels it is not helping. Even with daily naps, she awakens feeling very groggy and not rested, also admitting to increasing her red wine intake with her sleeping pill, hoping that could help her sleep at night.

She is slurring her speech somewhat and is very sluggish to respond to the questions. Her speech is slow, and her mentation is quite blunted.

Review of Systems

The patient's ROS is positive for unintentional weight gain, insomnia, lightheadedness, diaphoresis, SOB, clear productive cough, anorexia, and constipation. Her ROS is negative for fever, chills, headache, change in vision, trouble swallowing, hemoptysis, heart palpitations, abdominal pain, rectal bleeding, black or tarry stools, weakness, paresthesia, change in memory, syncope, or near syncope.

Relevant History

The patient has a past medical history significant for mitral valve stenosis secondary to rheumatic fever as a child, hyperlipidemia, osteoporosis, hyperparathyroidism that is being monitored, insomnia, age-related macular degeneration, and gout. She underwent a total abdominal hysterectomy at age 36 secondary to uterine fibroids and later bilateral salpingo-oophorectomy at age 50 secondary to benign ovarian masses. She has never used tobacco products, drinks 2 to 3 glasses of red wine after dinner, and does not use recreational or illicit drugs. Her diet consists of takeout fried chicken and microwaved frozen meals as she is a recent widow and states she has no one to cook for as she lives alone.

The patient's family history is significant for CAD and multiple myocardial infarcts in her mother, deceased at age 72, and in her brother, alive at age 72; her father, deceased at age 97 from CHF, pneumonia, and colon cancer; her sister, age 70, suffers from supraventricular tachycardia and gout. She has five adult children. Her three sons, ages 51, 48, and 46, are alive and all have HTN and hyperlipidemia. Her two daughters, ages 53 and 50 are alive and well with no known medical history.

ALLERGIES

No known drug allergies; no known food allergies, seasonal allergies related to pollen.

Medications

- Atorvastatin 40 mg QHS.
- Alendronate sodium 70 mg PO weekly.
- Vitamin D3 2000 IU PO BID.
- Colchicine 0.6mg PO QD.
- Lutein 40mg PO BID.
- Zolpidem 5mg PO QHS PRN insomnia.
- Loratadine 10mg PO QD PRN seasonal allergies.
- Triamcinolone acetonide nasal spray 55mcg spray, 1 spray each nostril BID PRN seasonal allergies.

Physical Examination

- *Vitals:* T 37.6°C (99.6°F), P 48, R 32, BP 174/98, HT 162.6 cm (64 in.), WT 73.5 kg (162 lb), BMI 27.8, SpO2 74% on room air.
- *General:* Elderly female who appears younger than stated age with slow, slurred speech, complaining of severe fatigue. Right-side dominant.
- *Psychiatric:* Altered mentation, oriented to person and place but not time.
- *Skin, Hair, and Nails:* Diaphoretic and clammy skin throughout, nailbeds of fingers and toes slightly cyanotic.
- *Head:* Normocephalic, atraumatic.
- *Eyes:* Sclera injected, nonicteric. Intact but sluggish EMOIs. PERRLA. No retinal hemorrhaging, AV nicking, optic disk cupping, papilledema.
- *ENT/Mouth:* Ear canals clear and patent with pale TMs bilaterally. No sinus tenderness. Lips slightly cyanotic. Dry mouth, patent oropharynx, uvula midline.
- *Neck:* Supple, (+) JVD bilaterally. No carotid thrills or bruits. Trachea midline, no goiter or lymphadenopathy.
- *Chest:* Tachypneic with retractions and accessory muscle use. Unable to take full deep breaths.
- *Lungs:* Audible crackling when patient speaks or exhales through mouth; crackles through all lung fields with wheezes at BL bases, extending to mid left lung. Does not clear with cough. Decreased tactile fremitus inferior lung fields bilaterally.
- *Heart:* Irregularly irregular rhythm, distant +S1/S2 with S3, IV/VI mitral murmur. Lateral displacement of PMI.
- *Peripheral Vascular:* 2+ pitting edema of BL UE extending proximally from fingers to elbows. 2+ pitting edema of BL LE extending proximally from toes to mid-tibias. Sluggish cap refill.
- *Abdomen:* Protuberant, soft, distant BS × 4. Slightly tender throughout all quadrants.
- *Neurologic:* Difficulty following commands. Tongue midline. Strength diminished and asymmetric throughout, R>L.

Clinical Discussion Questions

1. What is the differential diagnosis?

____

____

____

____

2. What is the most likely diagnosis? Why?

3. Demonstrate your understanding about the pathophysiology of the most likely diagnosis.

4. Should tests/imaging studies be ordered? Which ones? Why? Think about tests/imaging beyond the primary care setting as well.

5. What are the next appropriate steps in management?

6. What are the screening methods and diagnostic approaches for this diagnosis? Provide reference(s) with your response.

7. What are the pertinent ICD-10 and CPT (E/M) codes for this visit? Provide a short rationale.

8. What is the appropriate patient education topic for this case?

9. If not managed appropriately, what is/are the medical/legal concern(s) that may arise?

10. Think about interprofessional collaboration for this case. Provide a list of specialties or other disciplines and indicate what contribution these professionals might make to managing the patient.

BEDSIDE MANNER QUESTION

11. What would your communication style/approach be with this patient?

Answers available at courseconnect.springerpub.com.

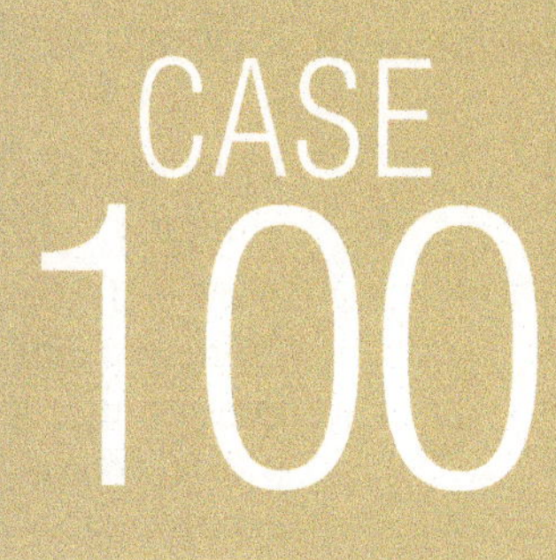

SUDDEN HEARING LOSS, GERIATRIC FEMALE

Chief Complaint

"I can't hear."

History of Present Illness

A 78-year-old White woman presents to the primary care clinic after waking up this morning with sudden hearing loss in her right ear. Patient denies ear pain, discharge from the ear, speech deficits, difficulty swallowing, nasal congestion, or sinus pressure. She denies ear pain and rates her pain as a 0 out of 10. Symptoms of hearing loss began today around 7:00 AM when the patient first awoke. Patient reports hearing loss in the right ear with normal hearing in the left ear. She denies a history of recent trauma, prior hearing loss, ringing in the ears, recent medication changes including starting any new medications, or exposure to loud music or noise.

Patient denies any history of ringing in her ears. She denies any constitutional symptoms, recent illness, sick contacts, trauma, or travel. She denies any difficulty with memory.

Review of Systems

The patient's ROS is positive for sudden hearing loss in the right ear. ROS is negative for neurologic, heart, lung, GI, GU, skin, or musculoskeletal symptoms.

Relevant History

The patient's medical history is significant for Graves disease, diagnosed at age 41 and treated with radioactive iodine. She subsequently developed hypothyroidism, which she continues to manage with levothyroxine 100 mcg QD. She experiences occasional tension headaches which she manages with OTC acetaminophen 650 mg Q6h PRN. Her only surgical history was a vaginal hysterectomy at age 62 with no complications and a tonsillectomy at age 8. For social history, the patient worked as an administrative assistant in her 20s and was a homemaker thereafter. She lives alone and has been a widow for 20 years.

Allergies

No known drug allergies; shellfish allergy.

Medications

- Levothyroxine 100 mcg PO QD for hypothyroidism.
- Acetaminophen 650 mg PO PRN Q6h for tension headache.

Physical Examination

- *Vitals* T 37.1°C (98.7°F), P 66, R 16, BP 120/78 mmHG, WT 54.4 kg (120 lb), HT 152.4 cm (60 in.), BMI 23.4.
- *General:* Well-appearing 78-year-old female in no acute distress, appears stated age.
- *Psychiatric:* Affect and mood are appropriate to setting.
- *Skin, Hair, and Nails:* No rashes noted, first-degree burn noted to cheeks, nose, and lips.
- *Head:* Normocephalic and atraumatic without tenderness, visible or palpable masses, depressions, or scarring. No evidence of bleeding or bruising. Hair is of normal texture and evenly distributed.

- *Eyes:* EOMI, PERRLA. Conjunctivae are clear without exudates or hemorrhage, and sclera are anicteric.
- *Ears:* Left ear pinna, tragus, and ear canal are nontender to palpation and without swelling. Left ear canal is clear without discharge. Left TM is pearly gray with light reflex intact and is not bulging or retracted. Hearing is intact with good acuity to whispered voice. Right ear pinna, tragus, and ear canal are nontender to palpation and without swelling. Right ear canal is completely occluded with cerumen. Right TM not visualized. Hearing is diminished with no acuity to whispered voice.
- *Nose:* Nasal mucosa is pink and moist. The nasal septum is midline. Nares patent bilaterally.
- *Throat/mouth:* Oral mucosa is pink and moist. Dentures are in place. Tongue normal in appearance without lesions and with good symmetrical movement. No buccal nodules or lesions are noted. The pharynx is normal in appearance without tonsillar tissue present.
- *Neck:* Supple with no adenopathy noted.
- *Neurologic:* A&O×3, gait intact.

Clinical Discussion Questions

1. What is the differential diagnosis?

2. What is the most likely diagnosis? Why?

3. Demonstrate your understanding about the pathophysiology of the most likely diagnosis.

4. Should tests/imaging studies be ordered? Which ones? Why? Think about tests/imaging beyond the primary care setting as well.

5. What are the next appropriate steps in management?

6. Review recent and credible research articles on about this diagnosis. Demonstrate your understanding of the different causes of conductive hearing loss and treatment approaches. Provide references with your response.

7. What are the pertinent ICD-10 and CPT (E/M) codes for this visit? Provide a short rationale.

8. What is the appropriate patient education topic for this case?

9. If not managed appropriately, what is/are the medical/legal concern(s) that may arise?

10. Think about interprofessional collaboration for this case. Provide a list of specialties or other disciplines and indicate what contribution these professionals might make to managing the patient.

BEDSIDE MANNER QUESTION

11. What would your communication style/approach be with this patient?

____

____

____

____

Answers available at courseconnect.springerpub.com.

SHORTNESS OF BREATH AND FATIGUE, GERIATRIC MALE

CASE 101

Chief Complaint

"Shortness of breath and fatigue."

History of Present Illness

A 71-year-old man visited his regular PCP complaining of SOB, particularly noticeable during outdoor activities like gardening and preparing his backyard for the winter. Additionally, he has been experiencing persistent fatigue toward the end of the day and feeling his heart beating faster during exercise. These symptoms have been gradually worsening over the last 6 months. He initially attributed symptoms to the natural effects of aging. His wife encouraged him to seek medical advice. He has not been monitoring his vital signs at home. He had COVID-19 2 months ago but currently reports no flu-like symptoms and he took a rapid antigen test at home that was negative. The patient was accompanied by his wife.

Review of Systems

The patient's ROS is positive for SOB, generalized weakness, palpitations, and fatigue. His ROS is negative for weight loss or gain, fever, chills, cough, expectorations, hemoptysis, flu-like symptoms, change in smell or taste, brain fog, confusion, headache, night sweats, orthopnea, swelling of the legs or abdomen, fainting, syncope, nausea, anxiety/depression, and environmental factors.

For the past 6 months, he has been experiencing increased fatigue toward the end of the day, as well as mild chest discomfort when he feels his heart palpitations. He denied the sensation of pressure or heaviness with his chest discomfort, and there is no radiation to his arms, neck, jaw, or back. He reported SOB and dizziness during physically demanding tasks, such as outdoor activities or playing with his grandchildren, but denied any chest pain. These symptoms were associated with slight weakness and reduced physical capacity compared to his usual state.

Relevant History

The patient has a personal medical history of systemic HTN treated with anti hypertensive drugs. His family history includes CAD in relatives above 65 years old, systemic HTN, and T2DM, but there is no family history of cancer or mental disease. In terms of lifestyle habits, he is a former smoker with a 20-year history of smoking, averaging 20 pack-years, and consumes three to four beers during the weekend. He maintains an active lifestyle—regularly walking and engaging in tasks in his backyard. He enjoys a varied and healthy diet, usually preparing home-cooked meals, and has a good appetite. He has been living with his wife for 45 years, has two children, four grandchildren, and several friends.

Allergies

No known drug allergies; no known food allergies.

Medications

Lisinopril 20 mg PO QD.

Physical Examination

- *Vitals:* T: 37.1°C (98.8°F), P 122 (regular), RR 24, BP 154/92, SaO_2 98%, WT 80 kg (176.37 lb), HT 170 cm (67 in.), BMI 27.62.

- *General:* Appears mildly fatigued, pale, and experiences SOB while moving on the examination table, no distress or diaphoresis.
- *Psychiatric:* The patient presents as calm, cooperative, and in a normal mood.
- *ENT/Mouth:* Normal, no cyanosis.
- *Neck:* Weak or delayed carotid upstroke, central venous pressure normal, no distention of the neck veins.
- *Lungs:* CTA bilaterally, no decreased breath sound intensity, expiratory phase longer, rales, crackles, or wheezing.
- *Heart:* Tachycardia with regular rhythm. A high pitched, diamond-shaped crescendo-decrescendo, mid-systolic ejection murmur, graded 3/6, was detected at the right upper sternal border, radiating to the carotid arteries.
- *Abdomen:* Normal, no swelling, hepatojugular reflux negative.
- *Musculoskeletal:* Normal, no Osler nodes.
- *Neurologic:* A&O.
- Dermatologic: No obvious lesions, warm and well-perfused, no signs of infection. No peripheral edema.

Clinical Discussion Questions

1. What is the differential diagnosis?

2. What is the most likely diagnosis? Why?

3. Demonstrate your understanding about the pathophysiology of the most likely diagnosis.

4. Should tests/imaging studies be ordered? Which ones? Why? Think about tests/imaging beyond the primary care setting as well.

5. What are the next appropriate steps in management?

6. Discuss the impact on quality of life, other associated conditions, risk factors, and treatment approach associated with this diagnosis. Provide references for your response.

7. What are the pertinent ICD-10 and CPT (E/M) codes for this visit? Provide a short rationale.

8. What is the appropriate patient education topic for this case?

9. If not managed appropriately, what is/are the medical/legal concern(s) that may arise?

10. Think about interprofessional collaboration for this case. Provide a list of specialties or other disciplines and indicate what contribution these professionals might make to managing the patient.

Bedside Manner Questions

11. What would your communication style/approach be with this patient?

12. If a patient or his wife is distressed by the diagnosis, what might offer support?

Answers available at courseconnect.springerpub.com.

LIST OF ABBREVIATIONS

2D	two-dimensional
2-h PG	2-hour plasma glucose
AAFP	American Academy of Family Practice
A1AT	alpha-1 antitrypsin
AAO	awake, alert, and oriented
AAP	American Academy of Pediatrics
AATD	alpha-1-antitrypsin deficiency
Ab	antibody
ABG	arterial blood gas
ABI	ankle-brachial index
ACA	Affordable Care Act
ACC	American College of Cardiology
ACE	angiotensin-converting enzyme
ACIP	Advisory Committee on Immunization Practices
ACLE	acute cutaneous lupus erythematosus
ACLS	advanced cardiac life support
ACS	acute coronary syndrome
ACTH	asdrenocorticotropic hormone
ADA	Americans with Disabilities Act
ADHD	attention-deficit hyperactivity disorder
ADLs	activities of daily living
A-Fib	atrial fibrillation
AFP	alpha-fetoprotein
AGEs	advanced glycation end products
AGS	American Geriatrics Society
AHA	American Heart Association
AHF	acute heart failure
AHI	Apnea-Hypopnea Index
AIH	autoimmune hepatitis
AIP	acute intermittent porphyria
AIS	adolescent idiopathic scoliosis
AKI	acute kidney injury
ALP	alkaline phosphatase
ALT	alanine transaminase
AMI	acute myocardial infarction
ANA	a-nuclear antibodies
ANC	absolute neutrophil count
AOM	acute otitis media
A&O	alert and oriented
A&O×3	alert and oriented to person, place, and time
A&O×4	alert and oriented to person, place, time, and event
AP	advanced placement
APA	American Psychological Association
APC	adenomatous polyposis coli
ARBs	angiotensin receptor blockers
ART	antiretroviral therapy
ASAP	as soon as possible
ASCVD	atherosclerotic cardiovascular disease
ASD	autism spectrum disorder
ASO	antistreptolysin O
ASQ-3	Ages & Stages Questionnaire, Third Edition
AST	aspartate aminotransferase
AUA	American Urological Association
AUD	alcohol use disorder
AUDIT-C	Alcohol Use Disorders Identification Test-Concise
AV	atrioventricular
aVL	augmented vector left
AVM	arteriovenous malformation
AVN	avascular necrosis
BASE	Brief Abuse Screen for the Elderly
BG	blood glucose
BID	twice daily
BL	bilateral
BLE	bilateral lower extremity
BMI	body mass index
BMP	basic metabolic panel

BNP	brain natriuretic peptide
BP	blood pressure
BPH	benign prostatic hypertrophy
BRAT	bananas, rice, applesauce, and toast
BRCA	breast cancer gene
BRUE	brief resolved unexplained event
BS	bowel sounds
BUN	blood urea nitrogen
BV	bacterial vaginosis
CAD	coronary artery disease
CBC	complete blood count
CBD	cannabidiol
CBT	cognitive behavioral therapy
CBT-I	cognitive behavioral therapy for insomnia
CCBs	calcium channel blockers
CCM	Chronic Care Model
CCP	cyclic citrullinated peptide
CCU	cardiac care unit
CD4	cluster of differentiation 4
CD8	cluster of differentiation 8
CDC	Centers for Disease Control and Prevention
CEA	carcinoembryonic antigen
CENTOR	Cough, Exudates, Nodes, Temperature, young OR old
CFS	cerebrospinal fluid
CFU	colony-forming unit
CGM	continuous glucose monitor
CHF	congestive heart failure
CHIP	Children's Health Insurance Program
CK	creatine kinase
CKD	chronic kidney disease
CKMB	creatine kinase myocardial band
CLIA	Clinical Laboratory Improvement Amendments
CM	Chiari malformations
CMAP	compound muscle action potential
CMP	comprehensive metabolic panel
CMV	cytomegalovirus
CN	cranial nerves
CNS	central nervous system
COMPLETES	Color, Other conditions, Mobility, Position, Lighting, Entire surface, Translucency, External auditory canal and auricle, Seal
COPD	chronic obstructive pulmonary disease
COVID-19	coronavirus disease 2019
COX	cyclooxygenase
CPAP	continuous positive airway pressure
CPF	chronic plantar fasciitis
CPS	Child Protective Services
CPT	Current Procedural Terminology
CPT (E/M)	Current Procedural Terminology (Evaluation and Management)
CRP	C-reactive protein
CSD	cat scratch disease
CSF	cerebrospinal fluid
CTA	clear to auscultation
CTS	carpal tunnel syndrome
CUP	cancer of unknown primary
CV	cardiovascular
CVA	cerebrovascular accident
CVD	coronary vascular disease
DAA	direct-acting antiviral
DASH	dietary approaches to stop hypertension
Dbili	direct bilirubin
DCCT	Diabetes Control and Complications Trial
DDx	differential diagnosis
DEXA	dual-energy x-ray absorptiometry
DGP	deamidated gliadin peptide
DJD	degenerative joint disease
DKA	diabetic ketoacidosis
DM	diabetes mellitus
DMT	disease-modifying therapy
DOH	Department of Health
DSM-5	*Diagnostic and Statistical Manual of Mental Disorders*, Fifth Edition
DSME	diabetes self-management, education
DSMS	diabetes self-management, support
DTaP	diphtheria and tetanus toxoids and acellular pertussis
DTR	deep tendon reflexes
DVT	deep vein thrombosis
EB	elementary body
EBV	Epstein–Barr virus
ED	emergency department
EEG	electroencephalogram
EF	ejection fraction
EGD	esophagogastroduodenoscopy
EGFR	epidermal growth factor receptor

eGFR	estimated glomerular filtration rate
EHR	electronic health records
EIA	enzyme immunoassay
EKG	electrocardiogram
ELISA	enzyme-linked immunoassay
EM	erythema multiforme
EMA	endomysial antibodies
EMDR	eye movement desensitization and reprocessing
EMG	electromyography
EMR	electronic medical records
EMS	emergency medical services
EMT	emergency medical technician
ENG	electronystagmography
ENP	emergency nurse practitioner
ENT	ear, nose, throat
EOM	extraocular movement
EOMI	extraocular movements intact
EP	electrophysiology
EPT	expedited partner therapy
ER	emergency room
ESBL	extended-spectrum beta-lactamase
ESLD	end-stage liver disease
ESR	erythrocyte sedimentation rate
ESWT	extracorporeal shock wave therapy
FABER	flexion, abduction, external rotation
FBS	fasting blood sugar
FDA	Food and Drug Administration
FEV1	forced expiratory volume in one second
FM	fibromyalgia
FMLA	Family Medical Leave Act
FOBT	fecal occult blood test
FODMAP	fermentable oligosaccharides, disaccharides, monosaccharides and polyols
FPG	fasting plasma glucose
FQHC	federally qualified health center
FROM	full range of motion
FSH	follicle-stimulating hormone
FSS	Functional Status Scale
FTA-ABS	fluorescent treponemal antibody absorbed
FVC	forced vital capacity
GABA	gamma-aminobutyric acid
GAD	general anxiety disorder
GAD-7	Generalized Anxiety Disorder 7-item
GAD 65	glutamic acid decarboxylase 65
GAS	group A streptococcus
GBM	glioblastoma multiforme
GC	gonococcal
GCA	giant cell arteritis
GCS	Glasgow Coma Scale
GE	gastroesophageal
GEJ	gastroesophageal junction
GERD	gastroesophageal reflux disease
GFD	gluten-free diet
GFR	glomerular filtration rate
GH	growth hormone
GI	gastrointestinal
GINA	Global Initiative for Asthma
GNAS1	guanine nucleotide binding protein, alpha stimulating
GP	gravidity and parity
GU	genitourinary
HAV	hepatitis A virus
HBcAb	hepatitis B core antibody
HBsAb	hepatitis B surface antibody
HBsAg	hepatitis B surface antigen
HC	head circumference
HCC	hepatocellular carcinoma
hCG	human chorionic gonadotropin
HCM	hypertrophic cardiomyopathy
Hct	hematocrit
HCTZ	hydrochlorothiazide
HCV	hepatitis C virus
HCVAb	hepatitis C virus antibodies
HD	hypokinetic dysarthria
HDL	high-density lipoprotein
HEADSS	Home, Education/Employment, Drug Use, Sexuality, and Self-harm
HEENT	head, eye, ear, nose, and throat
HER2	human epidermal growth factor receptor 2
HF	heart failure
HFMD	hand, foot, and mouth disease
Hgb	hemoglobin
Hgb A1C	hemoglobin A1C
HIV	human immunodeficiency virus
HLA	human leukocyte antigen
HNF	hepatocyte nuclear factor

HPI history of present illness
HPP hypokalemic periodic paralysis
HPV human papillomavirus
HR heart rate
HRA high-resolution anoscopy
HRT hormone replacement therapy
HS hidradenitis suppurativa
HSP Henoch-Schonlein purpura
HSV herpes simplex virus
HT height
HTN hypertension
IACS intra-articular corticosteroid
IBC inflammatory breast cancer
IBD inflammatory bowel disease
IBS irritable bowel syndrome
IBS-C irritable bowel syndrome with predominant constipation
IBS-D irritable bowel syndrome with predominant diarrhea
ICD International Classification of Diseases
I&D incision and drainage
ID infectious disease
IDSA Infectious Diseases Society of America
IDU injection drug use
IEP Individualized Education Program
IFA immunofluorescent antibody
IgA immunoglobulin A
IGF-1 insulin-like growth factor 1
IGIM intramuscular immunoglobulin
IgM immunoglobulin M
IL-15 interleukin-15
IM intramuscular
INS idiopathic nephrotic syndrome
IOP intraocular pressure
IPMDS International Parkinson and Movement Disorder Society
ISD intrinsic sphincteric deficiency
ITP idiopathic thrombocytopenic purpura
IU international unit
IUD intrauterine device
IV intravenous
JIA juvenile idiopathic arthritis
JIS juvenile idiopathic scoliosis
JRA juvenile rheumatoid arthritis
JVD jugular venous distention
KRAS Kirsten rat sarcoma
LABA/ICSI Long-acting beta-agonists and inhaled corticosteroids
LAD lymphadenopathy
LADA latent autoimmune diabetes of adulthood
LAMA long-acting muscarinic antagonist
LDH lactate dehydrogenase
LDL low-density lipoproteins
LES lower esophageal sphincter
LFTs liver function tests
LH luteinizing hormone
LLC lower limb cellulitis
LLQ left lower quadrant
LMP last menstrual period
LP lipoprotein
Lp(a) lipoprotein(a)
LPN licensed practical nurses
LROM limited range of motion
LS lumbar spine
LSM lifestyle modifications
LSW licensed clinical social worker
LVH left ventricular hypertrophy
LVN licensed vocational nurse
MA medical assistant
MALT mucosa-associated lymphoid tissue
MAS macrophage activation syndrome
MASLD metabolic dysfunction-associated steatotic liver disease
MCH mean corpuscular hemoglobin
MCHC mean corpuscular hemoglobin concentration
MCLS medial collateral ligament strain
MCN minimal-change nephropathy
MCV mean corpuscular volume
MD meningococcal disease
MDD major depressive disorder
MDI metered dose inhaler
MDS Movement Disorder Society
MG myasthenia gravis
MI myocardial infarction
MIRM *Mycoplasma pneumoniae*-induced rash and mucositis
MKPS medial knee plica syndrome
MMR measles, mumps, and rubella

MMRV	measles, mumps, rubella, and varicella
MMSE	Mini Mental State Examination
MODY	maturity-onset diabetes of youth
MRA	magnetic resonance angiography
MRSA	methicillin-resistant *Staphylococcus aureus*
MS	multiple sclerosis
MSCRAMMs	microbial surface components recognizing adhesive matrix molecules
MSI	microsatellite instability
MSM	men who have sex with men
MSSA	methicillin-sensitive *Staphylococcus aureus*
MSU	monosodium urate
MTLE	mesial (or medial) temporal lobe epilepsy
MVA	motor vehicle accident
NAAT	mucleic acid amplification test
NABS	normal active bowel sounds
NAC	non-*albicans Candida*
NAD	no acute distress
NAFLD	nonalcoholic fatty liver disease
NASH	nonalcoholic steatohepatitis
NCAT	normocephalic, atraumatic
NCS	nerve conduction study
NF	necrotizing fasciitis
NGSP	National Glycohemoglobin Standardization Program
NGU	nongonococcal urethritis
NICHQ	National Institute for Children's Health Quality
NO	nitric oxide
NOS	not otherwise specified
NP	nurse practitioner
NPO	nil per os
NSAIDs	nonsteroidal anti-inflammatory drugs
NSTEMI	non-ST segment elevation myocardial infarction
NSVD	normal spontaneous vaginal delivery
NT-BNP	N-terminal pro-B-type natriuretic peptide
NTLE	nocturnal temporal lobe epilepsy
NTND	Nontender nondistended
OA	osteoarthritis
OAB	overactive bladder
OAB-q	Overactive Bladder Questionnaire
OAB–V8	Overactive Bladder-Validated 8
OB-GYN	obstetrician-gynecologist
OCD	obsessive-compulsive disorder
OD	oculus dexter
ODD	oppositional defiant disorder
OE	otitis externa
OGTT	oral glucose tolerance test
OM	otitis media
OME	otitis media with effusion
OP	oropharynx
OR	operating room
OS	oculus sinister (left eye)
OSA	obstructive sleep apnea
OT	occupational therapy
OTC	over the counter
OU	O´culus uter´que (each eye)
PA	physician assistant
PACE	Program of All-Inclusive Care for the Elderly
PAD	peripheral artery disease
PAG	periaqueductal gray matter
PALM-COEIN	olyps, adenomyosis, leiomyoma, malignancy, and hyperplasia–coagulopathy, ovulatory dysfunction, endometrial, iatrogenic, and not otherwise classified
PBP-2a	penicillin-binding protein 2A
PCA	posterior circulating artery
PCMH	patient-centered medical home
PCOS	polycystic ovarian syndrome
PCP	primary care physician
PCR	polymerase chain reaction
PCV13	pneumococcal conjugate vaccine 13
PD	Parkinson disease
PDD	persistent depressive disorder
PE	pulmonary embolism
PEH	paraesophageal hernias
PERC	PE rule-out criteria
PERRL	pupil, equal, round, reactive (to), light
PERRLA	pupil, equal, round, reactive (to), light, accommodation
PES	peripheral electrical stimulation
PF	plantar flexion
PFS	patellofemoral syndrome
PHQ	Patient Health Questionnaire
PHQ2	Patient Health Questionnaire-2

PHQ-9	Patient Health Questionnaire-9
PI	phosphatidylinositol
PICU	pediatric ICU
PID	pelvic inflammatory disease
PKC	protein kinase C
PKD	polycystic kidney disease
PLT	platelets
PMI	point of maximal impulse
PMNs	polymorphonuclear neutrophils
PNS	primary nephrotic syndrome
PO	by mouth
POCBG	point-of-care blood sugar
POCUS	point-of-care ultrasound
PPIs	proton-pump inhibitors
PR	plaque rupture
PrEP	pre-exposure prophylaxis
PRN	as needed
PRP	platelet-rich plasma
PSA	prostate-specific antigen
PSGN	poststreptococcal acute glomerulonephritis
PSP	primary spontaneous pneumothorax
PT	physical therapist
PTA	peritonsillar abscess
PTH	parathyroid hormone
PT/INR	prothrombin time/international normalized ratio
PTNS	peripheral tibial nerve stimulation
PTSD	posttraumatic stress disorder
PTT	partial thromboplastin time
PVCs	premature ventricular contractions
PVD	peripheral venous disease
QD	daily
QHS	every night at bedtime
QID	four times daily
QTC	QT interval corrected
RA	rheumatoid arthritis
RAAS	renin–angiotensin–aldosterone system
RAI	radioactive iodine therapy
RAMs	rapid alternating movements
RB	reticulate body
RBC	red blood cell
RBS	random blood sugar
RDW	red cell distribution width
RF	rheumatoid factor
RICE	Rest, Ice, Compression, and Elevation
RIDT	rapid influenza diagnostic test
RLQ	right lower quadrant
RMSF	Rocky Mountain spotted fever
RNA	ribonucleic acid
ROM	range of motion
ROS	review of systems
RPR	rapid plasma reagin
RR	regular rate
RRMS	relapsing remitting multiple sclerosis
RRR	regular rate and rhythm
RSR	regular sinus rhythm
RSV	respiratory syncytial virus
RT-PCR	reverse transcription polymerase chain reaction
RUQ	right upper quadrant
RZV	recombinant zoster vaccine
SA	sinoatrial
SAD	seasonal affective disorder
SARS-CoV-2	Severe acute respiratory syndrome coronavirus 2
SB	sickle beta
SC	sickle cell
SCARED	Screen for Childhood Anxiety-Related Emotional Disorders
SCC	staphylococcal chromosome cassette
SCD	sickle cell disease
SCQ	Social Communication Questionnaire
SG	specific gravity
SGL	same-gender loving
SGLT2	sodium glucose cotransporter 2
SHBG	sex hormone binding globulin
SIRS	systemic inflammatory response syndrome
SJIA	systemic juvenile idiopathic arthritis
SJS	Stevens-Johnson syndrome
SLE	systemic lupus erythematosus
SLR	straight leg raise
SNHL	sensorineural hearing loss
SNRI	serotonin and norepinephrine reuptake inhibitors
SOAP	Subjective, Objective, Assessment, and Plan
SOB	shortness of breath

SRCs sports-related concussions
SSRIs selective serotonin reuptake inhibitors
SSS Symptom Severity Scale
SSTI skin and soft tissue infection
STAT immediately
STD sexually transmitted disease
STEMI ST-segment elevation myocardial infarction
STI sexually transmitted infection
SUD substance use disorder
T1DM type 1 diabetes mellitus
T2DM type 2 diabetes mellitus
TAH/BSO total abdominal hysterectomy with bilateral salpingo-oophorectomy
TAPS transcutaneous afferent patterned stimulation
TB tuberculosis
TBI traumatic brain injury
Tbili total bilirubin
TBUT tear break-up time
TCAs tricyclic antidepressants
Tdap tetanus, diphtheria, acellular pertussis
TEACCH Treatment and Education of Autistic and Related Communication Handicapped Children
TG transglutaminase
THC tetrahydrocannabinol
TIAs transient ischemic attacks
TIBC total iron binding capacity
TID three times a day
TM tympanic membrane
TMJ temporomandibular joint
TMN thin membrane nephropathy
TMP–SMX trimethoprim–sulfamethoxazole
TPO thyroid peroxidase
TPP thyrotoxic periodic paralysis
TRT testosterone replacement therapy
TSH thyroid-stimulating hormone
TSH-R thyroid-stimulating hormone receptor
TSI thyroid-stimulating immunoglobulin
TTE transthoracic echocardiogram
TTG tissue transglutaminase
TTP thrombotic thrombocytopenic purpura
TV trichomonas vaginalis
UA urine analysis
UAhCG urine analysis human chorionic gonadotropin
UC ulcerative colitis
UE upper extremity
URI upper respiratory infection
US ultrasound
USPSTF United States Preventive Services Task Force
UTI urinary tract infection
UV ultraviolet
UVB ultraviolet B
VCUG voiding cystourethrogram
VDRL Venereal Disease Research Laboratory
VSD ventricular septal defect
VSS vulvovaginal sensory syndrome
VVC vulvovaginal candidiasis
WBC white blood cell
WHO World Health Organization
WNL within normal limit
WT weight

INDEX